EKG/ECG

INTERPRETATION MADE SIMPLE

A Practical Approach to Passing the ECG/EKG Portion of NCLEX

Amanda Caldwell

Copyright

The Information contained in this book is for training nursing students for NCLEX only. This information is meant to be a supplement to a more thorough training class. The information is only considered accurate up to the date of publication.

Disclaimer This Book contains information that is intended to help the readers pass the ECG Portion of their NCLEX test. It is presented as general training on health care. While we try to keep the information up-to-date and correct, there are no representations or warranties, express or implied, about the completeness, accuracy, reliability, suitability or availability with respect to the information, products, services, or related graphics contained in this Book for any purpose.

Printed in the United States of America

Quick Medical Guide Publishers

USA | CANADA

Contents

Chapter 3

Chapter 4

Chapter 5

Chapter 6

Chapter 7

Introduction

The electrocardiogram (ECG) also known as Electrokardiogram (EKG) is one of the most useful diagnostic tests in emergency medicine. It is an easy and inexpensive test that is used routinely in the assessment of patients with chest pain. The ECG is the cornerstone for making the diagnosis of cardiac ischemia and is used for making decisions about eligibility for thrombolytic therapy.

Most books use ECG and EKG interchangeably and they both mean the same thing. The K in EKG means "Kardio" which is a German word for "Cardio."

To avoid misinterpreting the ECG, the clinician must have a systematic approach. This book is designed to guide the learner through a stepwise approach to ECG interpretation. Specific questions and answers of ECG portion of NCLEX are included at the end.

Chapter 1

Understanding the Principles Of Cardiac Electrophysiology And ECG Interpretation

For the heart to work effectively, the atria and the ventricles must be activated rapidly and sequentially. Rapid activation is important in order to activate as much myocardium simultaneously as possible; the more myocardium contracting at the same time the more efficient the pumping mechanism. Sequential activation implies that the atria are activated first and they fill the ventricles with adequate volumes of blood, before ventricular contraction commences. To coordinate these two tasks, the heart has an electrical conduction system composed of specialized myocardial cells (henceforth referred to as conduction cells).

These cells form bundles of fibers which act as electrical cords that spread the action potential rapidly and sequentially to contractile myocardium in the atria and the ventricles. When contractile myocardium receives the action potential, it is activated and contracts. **Figure 1** illustrates relevant components of the conduction system, the heart and the classical ECG waveforms.

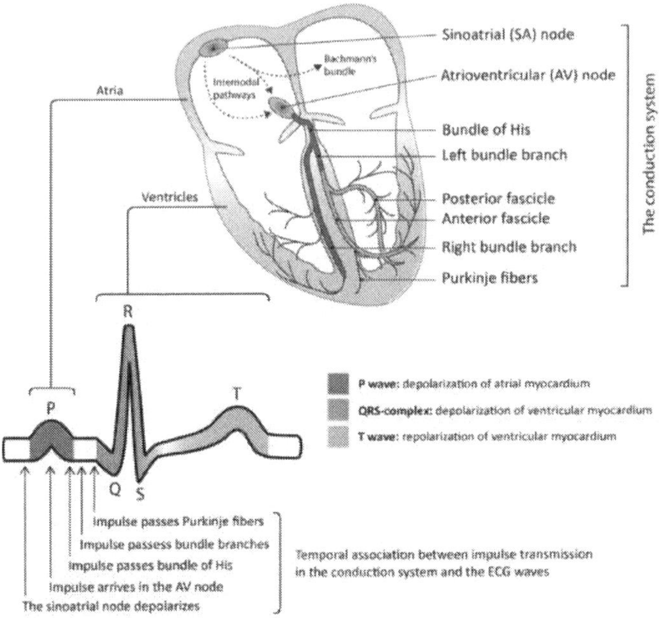

Figure 1. The cardiac cycle starts when cells in the sinoatrial node discharges an action potential that spreads as an electrical impulse through the atria and – via the atrioventricular node – to the ventricles. As the impulse spreads through the myocardium, it activates the cells which respond by contracting. The action potential generates electrical currents which gives rise to the classical ECG waveforms presented

here.

Activation of the atrial is reflected as the P-wave and activation of the ventricles results in the QRS complex. The T-wave reflects the recovery (repolarization) of the ventricles. Note that the ECG rarely shows atrial recovery (repolarization) since it coincides with ventricular depolarization (i.e QRS complex), which has much stronger electrical potentials.

Types of Cell in Electrocardiology

For the purpose of this discussion it is important to distinguish between two main types of cardiac cells:

- **Conduction cells** form the fiber networks that sprout into the myocardium and disseminate the action potential. These cells have virtually no contractile function.
- **Contractile myocardial cells** carry out the actual contraction but are also capable of transmitting the action potential, albeit at a much lower speed than the conduction cells. The terms *contractile myocardium*, *myocardium* or

simply *myocardial cell*, refer to this cell type and these terms are used interchangeably.

Cardiac cell architecture

In contrast to skeletal muscle, cardiac cells display a branch-like morphology. As illustrated in **Figure 2** below all cardiac cells are connected, both electrically and mechanically, along their long axis. This cell architecture is referred to as a **syncytium**, which implies that the entire network of cells functions as one unit.

It follows that if one cell in the syncytium is activated, it will activate all cells downstream (provided that they are excitable). The connections between the cells are termed **intercalated discs**. The intercalated disc is composed of cell membrane proteins that connects adjacent cells both mechanically and electrically. The electrical connection is established by **gap junctions**, which are proteins that forms channels between the cell membranes. Electrically charged ions can flow between cells through the gap junctions. It follows that the action potential can spread from one cell to the next using this route.

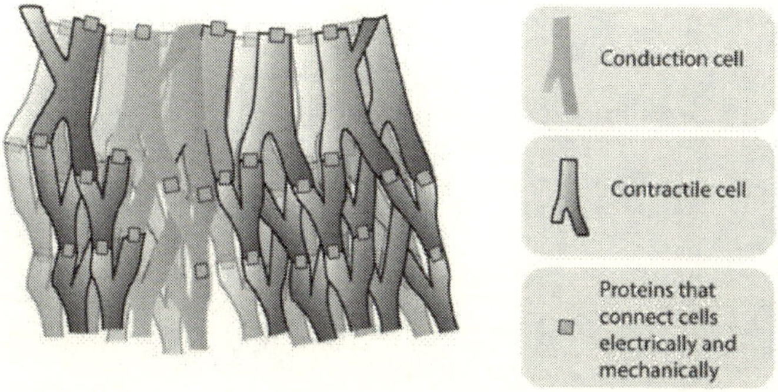

Figure 2. Schematic illustration of the myocardial syncytium. Note the branched cell structure and the connections between the cells.

Understanding the cardiac action potential

The *action potential* includes a *depolarization (activation)* followed by a *repolarization (recovery)*. As mentioned above, the cardiac cycle starts when the sinoatrial node discharges the first action potential, which then spreads through the myocardium like a wave front in water. Specific ion channels located on the cell membranes open and close during de- and repolarization, such that ions (Na^+ [sodium], K^+

[potassium], Ca2+ [calcium]) can flow between the intra- and extracellular compartment. Thus, the action potential involves movement of ions – which are charged particles – and therefore the action potential generates an electrical current. **Figure 3** (below) shows the appearance of the action potential in myocardial cells (the action potential will be discussed in detail in the next chapter.

Note that the terms ***electrical impulse***, ***impulse*** and ***impulse wave*** are used interchangeably to refer to the wave-like spread of the action potential in the myocardium.

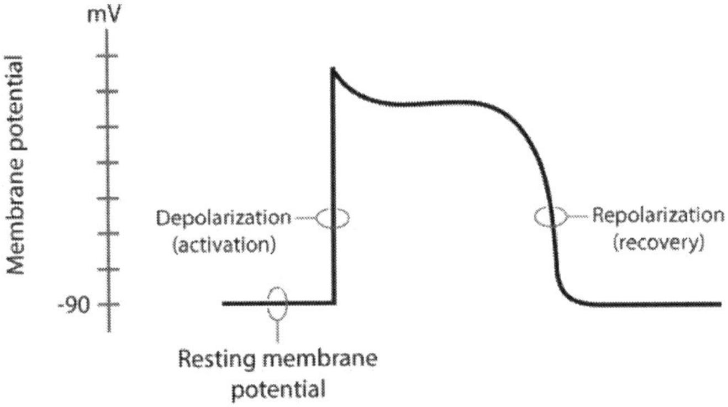

Figure 3. The action potential of contractile cells. Inactive (resting) myocardial cells have a resting membrane potential of -90 mV. Upon stimulation, the

cell depolarizes and a rapid increase in the membrane potential is noted. The cell returns to its resting state by repolarizing. These concepts are discussed in detail in the next chapter.

Cardiac electromechanical coupling

Depolarization activates the myocardial cells and induces cellular processes that lead to cell contraction. The spread of an electrical impulse is therefore directly coupled to a mechanical event (this is referred to as **electromechanical coupling**). Because there is an abundance of ions in the tissues and fluids surrounding the heart - and indeed in the entire human body – the electrical currents generated in the heart are transmitted all the way to the skin, where they can be recorded using electrodes.

Electrocardiography is the art of recording and interpreting the electrical potentials generated in the myocardium. The electrocardiograph presents these electrical events in a diagram referred to as electrocardiogram (ECG).

The electrical potentials generated by components of

the conduction system (sinoatrial node, atrioventricular node, bundle of His, Purkinje fibers) are too small to be detected using surface (skin) electrodes. Hence, the ECG only presents activity of contractile atrial and ventricular myocardium. This is unfortunate because the conduction system plays a pivotal role in cardiac function and certainly ECG interpretation. Luckily, it is almost always possible to draw conclusions about the conduction system based on the visible ECG waveforms and rhythm. In some instances, however, invasive electrophysiological studies (recording of electrical activity from inside the heart using catheters equipped with electrodes) is necessary.

The electrical conduction system of the heart

The sinoatrial node (SA node)

The sinoatrial node is a small oval structure located near the entrance of the superior vena cava in the right atrium (Figure 1). The sinoatrial node consists of highly specialized cells with a distinct ability to depolarize spontaneously, without being stimulated. Thus, the cells of the sinoatrial node are capable of spontaneously discharging an action potential. This ability to depolarize spontaneously is referred to as automaticity. The cells of the sinoatrial node have an intrinsic rate (frequency) of depolarization at approximately 70 times per minute (which results in 70 heart beats per minute). The sinoatrial node is often referred to as the primary pacemaker of the heart.

The rate of spontaneous depolarization in the sinoatrial node is modified by the autonomic nervous system. Sympathetic stimulation increases the rate whereas parasympathetic stimulation lowers the rate. Hence, heart rate increases as sympathetic tone is increased and heart rate decreases as parasympathetic tone increases. The heart rate at any given instant depends on the balance between sympathetic and parasympathetic activity. Sympathetic activity dominates during physical exercise, whereas parasympathetic activity dominates during rest.

Secondary (latent) pacemakers

The sinoatrial node is the primary pacemaker of the heart. However, there are additional structures that possess automaticity and thus the ability to serve as the heart's pacemaker. These structures are as follows:

- **Parts of the atrial myocardium**: There are clusters of atrial myocardial cells located around the crista terminalis, the entrance of the coronary sinus and the inferior vena cava, as well as cells around the mitral and tricuspid valves, which possess automaticity. These cells are not conduction cells per se; they are actually contractile cells which possess automaticity. Thus, automaticity is not exclusive to cells of the conduction system.
- **Myocardium surrounding the atrioventricular (AV) node**: It is a common misconception that the atrioventricular (AV) node possesses automaticity, because there is no compelling evidence for that. There is, however, evidence that cell clusters surrounding the

AV node possess automaticity. This automaticity will still – despite what has just been stated – be referred to as automaticity of the AV node in order to facilitate understanding.

- **The His-Purkinje network**: The bundle of His and the entire Purkinje network possess automaticity.

The observant reader may have noticed that the ventricular myocardium does not possess automaticity, and this is important to note as we shall see in later chapters.

Thus, the heart has four pacemakers (the sinoatrial node; parts of atrial myocardium; myocardium around the AV node; the His-Purkinje network). The reason that the sinoatrial node is the primary pacemaker is simply because it has the highest intrinsic rate of spontaneous depolarization (i.e the fastest automaticity). Heart rhythm is directed by the fastest pacemaker (i.e the structure with the highest rate of spontaneous depolarization) because that pacemaker will depolarize before the competing pacemakers and reset them before they discharge an action potential.

Studying the clinical aspects of automaticity

The sinoatrial node may become dysfunctional and fail to depolarize. Failure to depolarize may be intermittent, or persistent for longer periods or even permanent. This could potentially result in cardiac arrest but it rarely does, because absence of sinoatrial impulses will allow for one of the other pacemakers to establish a heart rhythm.

This behavior is the reason why the other pacemakers are often referred to as latent pacemakers. The intrinsic rate of spontaneous depolarization in the latent pacemakers is highest in the atrial myocardium and lowest in the Purkinje fibers. Thus, automaticity appears to decline gradually with the distance from the sinoatrial node. This means that if the sinoatrial node fails to depolarize, it is most likely that a salvaging rhythm will be established by atrial myocardium. Should the atrial myocardium also fail, then it is most likely that the cells around the atrioventricular node will take over the rhythm.

As a last resort there is an extensive network of Purkinje fibers, starting in the bundle of His, which can establish a rhythm. This succession, from the sinoatrial node to the Purkinje fibers, is referred to as **pacemaker hierarchy**. **Figure 4** displays the pacemaker hierarchy.

It should be noted that the automaticity discussed above is normal automaticity, which only occurs in the sinoatrial node and the latent pacemakers. However, there is also abnormal automaticity, which can arise anywhere in the heart, including in ventricular myocardium.

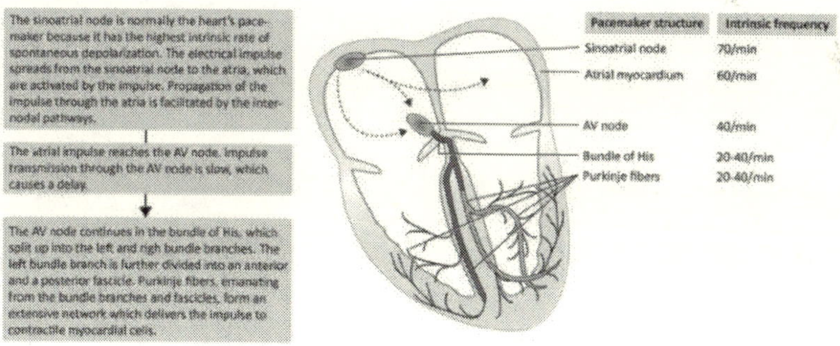

Figure 4. Overview of the electrical impulse during a

cardiac cycle (left hand side) and the pacemaker hierarchy (right hand side). All pacemaker structures are capable of spontaneous depolarization (automaticity), and can therefore serve as the heart's pacemaker. The rate of spontaneous depolarization is highest in the sinoatrial node, which is why it is the primary pacemaker.

Impulse transmission (conduction, propagation)

The cells of the conduction system have virtually no contractile function. Conduction cells are merely responsible for spreading the depolarization rapidly and synchronously to the contractile cells, so that they can contract in concert. However, there are fewer conduction cells than contractile cells, which implies that conduction cells only communicate with a portion of the contractile myocardium.

The remaining contractile cells, which do not communicate directly with conduction cells, depend on other contractile cells to obtain the electrical impulse. Recall that all cells in the heart are connected, both mechanically and electrically and this enables the electrical impulse to spread from one cell to the next. However, impulse transmission between contractile myocardial cells is considerably slower than transmission through the conduction fibers.

Atrial impulse transmission

The conduction system is vaguely defined in the atria, as compared with the ventricles which boasts with distinct conduction structures such as the bundle of His and the bundle branches. There are, however, three rather distinct fiber bundles which appear to serve as the conduction system of the atria. These bundles transmit the atrial impulse at a speed of 1 m/s and they are referred to as the internodal pathways. One of these is Bachmann's bundle, which conducts the impulse from the right to the left atrium. Refer to Figure 1 (above).

The atrioventricular conduction system

The atrioventricular node (AV node)

The atrioventricular (AV) node is the bridge between the atria and the ventricles. It is located in the atrial septum and normally the only connection between the atria and ventricles (Figure 1). The AV node receives the atrial impulse and delays it before conducting it to the ventricles. The delay is due to the slow conduction through the atrioventricular node. The purpose of the slow conduction is to give the atria adequate time to fill the ventricles with blood, before ventricular contraction commences.

The bundle of His

The atrioventricular node continues in the bundle of His which splits up in the left bundle branch and the right bundle branch. These bundles successively branch into finer bundles and ultimately Purkinje fibers which sprout into the myocardium. Note that the left bundle branch splits into an anterior and a posterior fascicle.

The Purkinje fibers

Impulse transmission in the Purkinje network is very fast (4 m/s). The Purkinje fibers run mainly through the endocardium where they deliver the depolarizing impulse to contractile myocardial cells. Some Purkinje fibers extend deeper into the myocardium (rarely deeper than a third of the wall's thickness). This means that activation of the ventricles (except from the septum) starts in the endocardium and spreads towards the epicardium (**Figure 5**). The rapid impulse transmission in the Purkinje network allows virtually all ventricular myocardium to be activated simultaneously. As noted above, when the impulse is delivered to the contractile myocardial cells, the subsequent impulse transmission takes place from one contractile cell to the next, which is much slower (0.4 m/s).

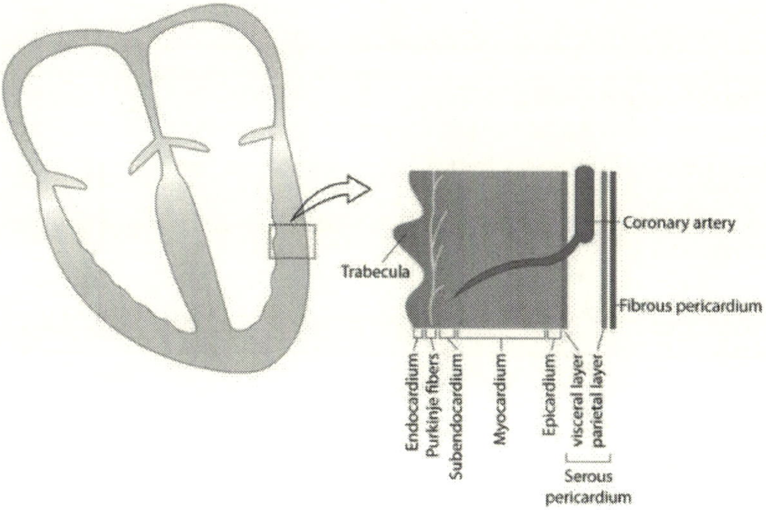

Figure 5. Schematic figure of the ventricular wall.

Note that the term myocardium is often used to refer to all layers.

Influences of the autonomic nervous system

The vagus nerve provides the heart with parasympathetic fibers. These fibers primarily innervate the sinoatrial node and the atrioventricular node. Increased vagal tone leads to slowed automaticity in the sinoatrial node and slowed conduction through the atrioventricular node. This leads to lower heart rate (and a negligble increase in the delay in the atrioventricular node). Intensive vagal activity may actually inhibit sinoatrial activity to the extent that no impulses are generated and this may lead to syncope (fainting). As discussed above, latent pacemakers will awake and take over generation of action potentials until the sinoatrial node recovers.

Sympathetic fibers innervate the entire heart, both the conduction system and contractile myocardium. The fibers run along the blood vessels and are particularly dense in ventricular myocardium. Sympathetic stimulation leads to increased excitability in all cells. This means that increased sympathetic activity results in increased heart rate (by increasing automaticity in the sinoatrial node), increased contractile force and increased speed of impulse conduction.

Definition of heart rhythm

A rhythm is defined as three consecutive heart beats displaying (more or less) identical waveforms on the ECG. The similarity of the waveforms indicates that their origin is the same. The sinoatrial node is the heart's pacemaker under normal circumstances and the rhythm is referred to as *sinus rhythm*. Although it is not possible to discern the electrical potentials of the sinoatrial node itself, there are indirect evidence from the ECG that confirm the origin of the rhythm.

Should any structure outside of the sinoatrial node discharge an action potential that results in myocardial depolarization, that structure is referred to as **ectopic focus** and the beat is called an **ectopic beat**.

An **ectopic rhythm** occurs when three or more consecutive heart beats originate from an ectopic focus. If an ectopic rhythm is a replacement for the normal sinus rhythm, it is referred to as **escape rhythm**.

In conclusion, The cardiac cycle begins when the sinoatrial node discharges an action potential that spreads through the heart. The action potential spreads in the form of an electrical impulse, by cell-to-cell transmission of the depolarization. The impulse spreads via the internodal pathways and Bachmann's bundle in the atria. It is then delayed briefly in the atrioventricular node before it is rapidly disseminated – via the His-Purkinje network – through the ventricular myocardium. The contraction starts when contractile cells receive the impulse.

The action potential consists of a depolarization (activation) and a repolarization (recovery). This process includes rapid changes in the membrane potential, which is a consequence of ions flowing across the cell membrane. Flow of ions is equal to an electrical current and the electrical activity of atrial and ventricular myocardium is recorded and analysed by electrodes placed on the skin. ECG interpretation is all about deciphering these electrical currents.

You can study the Wiggers diagram below. It displays the association between the ECG, pressure and volume in the heart during the cardiac cycle.

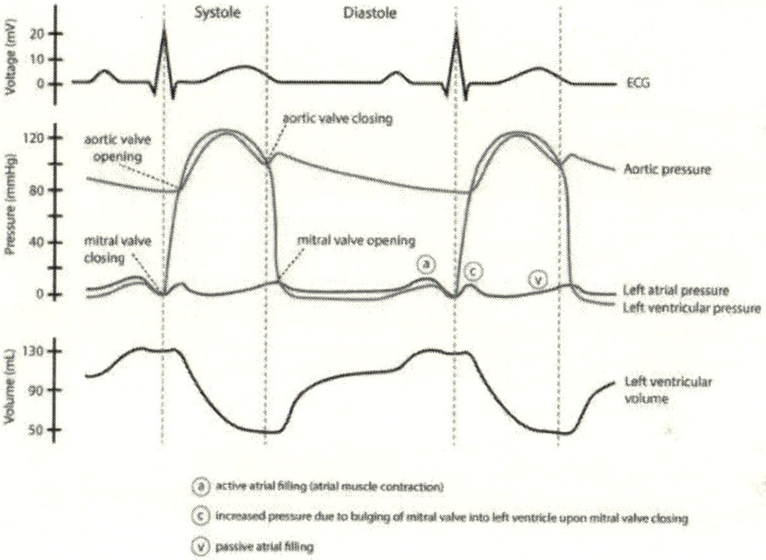

Figure 6. A Wiggers diagram is a standard diagram used in cardiac physiology to illustrate the association between aortic pressure, ventricular pressure, atrial pressure, volumes and ECG waveforms.

Chapter 2

Cardiac Electrophysiology: action potential, automatic and electrical vectors

The action potential includes a **depolarization** (activation) followed by a **repolarization** (recovery). The action potential occurs in all cardiac cells but its appearance varies depending on cell type. During de- and repolarization ions (Na+ [sodium], K+ [potassium] and Ca2+ [calcium]) flows back and forth across the cell membrane. Because ions are electrically charged, their movement generates an electrical current. This means that propagation (spread) of the action potential is equal to spread of an electrical current.

All tissues and fluids surrounding the heart have an abundance of ions, which means that they can act as electrical conductors. Consequently, the electrical currents generated in the myocardium are transmitted all the way to the skin, where they can be detected by electrodes. The electrocardiograph (ECG machine) records and processes these electrical currents and presents them as the electrocardiogram (ECG).

As mentioned earlier, the electrical potentials of the conduction system are much too minute to be detected by skin electrodes; the ECG presents electrical activity of atrial and ventricular myocardium.

Automaticity of pacemaker cells

The automaticity of the cells in the sinoatrial node is explained by the fact that these cells start leaking sodium (Na+) into the cell as soon as they return to their resting state (Figure 1). As sodium leaks into the cell, the cell membrane gradually becomes more positive. When the membrane potential reaches its threshold −40 mV, the action potential is triggered and the cell depolarizes. At −40 mV voltage gated calcium (Ca2+) channels open so that calcium flows into the cell and cause the depolarization.

Subsequently, outward directed potassium (K+) channels open which results in repolarization of the cell. The cycle then repeats itself (**Figure 1**). Note that the leakage of sodium during the resting phase is called **pacemaker potential**.

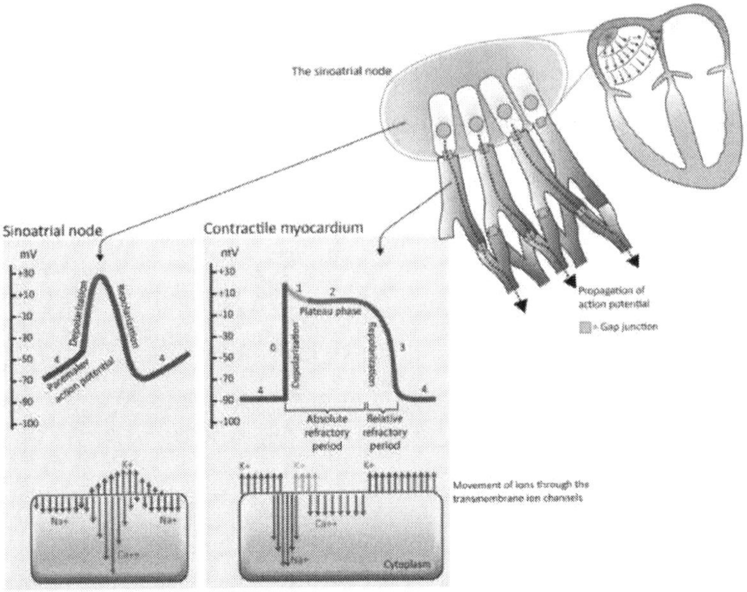

Figure 1. The action potential in the sinoatrial node and in contractile myocardial cells. Phase 4 of the action potential in the sinoatrial node is called 'pacemaker potential', because it is responsible for the spontaneous repetitive depolarization.

The depolarization spreads from the sinoatrial node to the atrial and ventricular myocardium. Propagation of the action potential is possible because all cardiac cells are electrically interconnected by gap junctions (Figure 1). Gap junctions are protein channels that connect the cell membranes of adjacent cells and enable flow of ions between cells. This means that the action potential spreads from one cell to another via gap junctions.

The density of gap junctions within the Purkinje network is very high, which explains the rapid impulse transmission in the network. Cells of the atrioventricular node, on the other hand, have very low density of gap junctions, which explains the slow impulse conduction through the atrioventricular node. Transmission of the action potential between contractile myocardial cells is also slow, owing to the scarcity of gap junctions between them.

The contractile cells, unlike cells of the sinoatrial node, display a true resting potential (phase 4), which is around -90 mV. These cells must be stimulated in order to evoke an action potential. Upon stimulation, sodium (Na+) channels open which causes a rapid influx of sodium and depolarizes the cell. Contractile cells start to contract a few milliseconds after start of the depolarization and they starts relaxing a few milliseconds after the repolarization is completed. The duration of the action potential is approximately 0.20 seconds in atrial myocardium and 0.3 seconds in ventricular myocardium (**Figure 1**).

The action potential in contractile cells

The phases are also illustrated in **Figure 1** (above).

- **Phase 4 (resting phase)**: Only potassium (K+) channels are open during the resting phase and efflux (outward flow) of potassium establishes a negative resting membrane potential (approximately −90 mV).
- **Phase 0 (depolarization)**: Upon stimulation, rapid depolarization occurs via influx (inward flow) of sodium (Na+) and the cell becomes positively charged (approximately 20 mV).
- **Phase 1 (early repolarization)**: During this phase, another type of potassium (K+) channels open and a brief efflux of potassium repolarizes the cell slightly.
- **Phase 2 (plateau phase)**: Almost

simultaneous with the opening of potassium channels in phase 1, persistent calcium (Ca2+) channels open whereby calcium flows into the cell. The influx of calcium is steady and give rise to the plateau phase whose long duration explains why the vast majority of the ventricular myocardium contracts simultaneously (at some point during the contraction).

- **Phase 3 (repolarization)**: Calcium (Ca2+) channels close and potassium (K+) channels open again and the efflux of potassium repolarizes the cell.

Absolute and relative refractory periods during the action potential

During the greater part of the action potential the myocardial cell is **absolute refractory** to stimulation, meaning that an additional stimulus cannot trigger a new action potential, regardless of the intensity of the stimulus. The absolute refractory period is followed by a **relative refractory period**, during which a strong stimulation may trigger a new action potential. The absolute and relative refractory periods are displayed in **Figure 1** (above) and **Figure 2** (below).

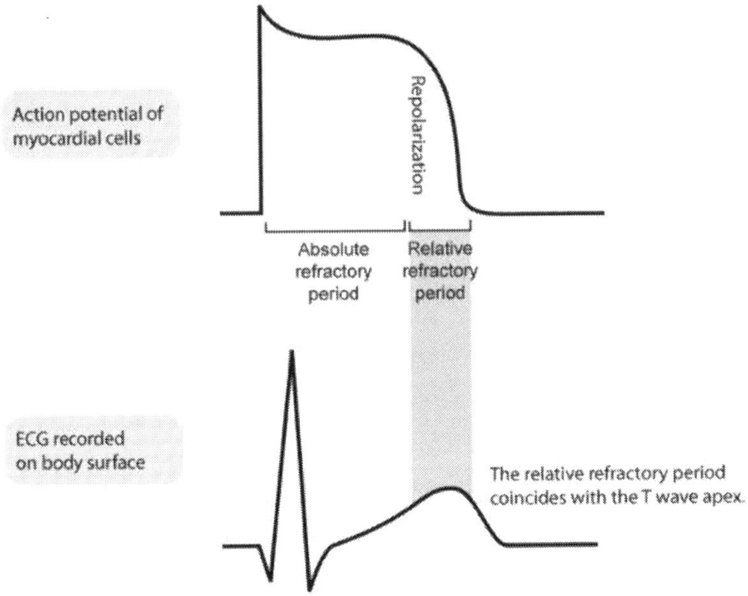

Figure 2. Absolute and relative refractory periods during the action potential.

As seen in **Figure 2** the relative refractory period coincides with the T-wave apex. This phase has traditionally been described as a vulnerable phase during the cardiac cycle, because electrical stimulation during this phase may evoke another action potential which can lead to potentially life-threatening ventricular arrhythmias (ventricular fibrillation).

This occurs occasionally in clinical practice. The stimulus is typically a premature ventricular beat (i.e an ectopic beat from within the ventricles) or inappropriate stimulation from an artificial pacemaker. When such a ventricular depolarization is superimposed on the T-wave, it is said that an **R-on-T phenomenon** has occurred. However, it should be noted that R-on-T phenomenon are very common and the risk of ventricular fibrillation is negligible, unless there is electrical instability in the ventricles (such as during acute myocardial infarction). Figure 3 (below) shows two cases of R-on-T phenomenon.

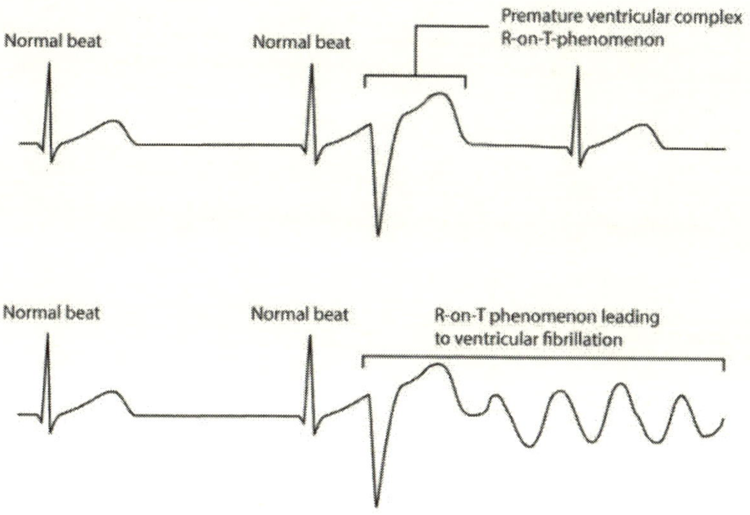

Figure 3. R-on-T phenomenon

What does the ECG show?

Figure 4 below shows the classical ECG waveforms. The first deflection (henceorth called wave) is the **P-wave** which represents activation (depolarization) of the atria. The repolarization of the atria is usually not visible because it occurs simultaneously as the activation (depolarization) of the ventricles, which generates substantially larger electrical potentials and therefore dominates that moment in the cardiac cycle. Ventricular depolarization is visible as the **QRS complex**. The QRS complex consists of three waves: Q, R and S. Differences in the direction of these waves are due to changes in the direction of the electrical impulse during ventricular depolarization. The **T-wave** represents repolarization of the ventricles.

Note the straight line between the P-wave and the QRS complex (Figure 4). This line is referred to as the **PR segment** and it represents the impulse delay in the atrioventricular node.

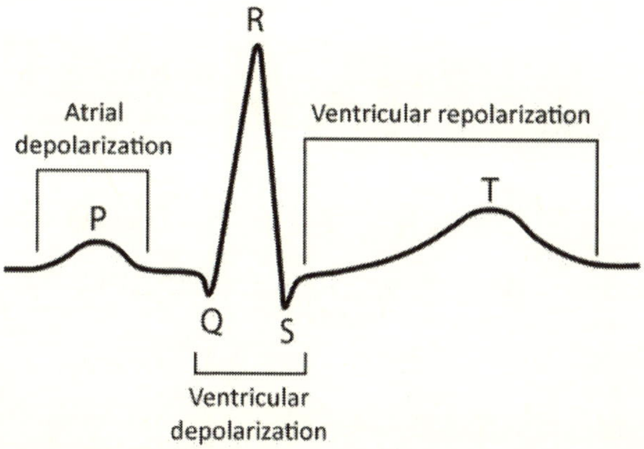

Figure 4. The classical ECG curve and the events reflected on it. The ECG curve above displays a QRS complex consisting of Q-, R- and S-wave. Even if one or two waves would be missing from the QRS complex, it would still be referred to as the QRS complex.

It is fundamental to know the genesis of these waveforms and this requires knowledge of the electrical vectors that exist during the cardiac cycle. Vector theory is a rather complex matter, which is why the discussion below will exclude overly complicated aspects and focus on the main electrical vectors and how they impact the ECG curve.

Electrical vectors

A vector is a physical quantity which has both magnitude and direction in space. Movement of electrically charged particles – which occur during spread of the cardiac action potential – generates an electrical vector. The depolarization propagates through the myocardium similar to the spread of a wave front in water. At any given instant in time there are numerous small depolarizing wave fronts that propagate through the myocardium.

In order to understand how an electrical vector generates a wave on the ECG curve, it is crucial to understand how ECG leads function. Note that the ECG leads will be discussed in detail in the next chapter; here we only mention aspects relevant to electrical vectors. The electrocardiograph (ECG machine) uses two electrodes to calculate one ECG curve (**Figure 5**). This is done by comparing the electrical potentials detected by each of the electrodes. One electrode is defined as positive (also called exploring electrode) and the other is negative (also called reference electrode). The electrocardiograph compares the electrical potentials detected by the exploring electrode and the reference electrode. The machine is constructed such that a vector heading towards the exploring electrode yields a positive deflection (wave) on the ECG curve. A vector heading away from the exploring electrode yields a negative wave (**Figure 5**).

It is traditionally taught that the exploring electrode is the one "viewing" the heart, and this notion actually facilitates ECG interpretation. Later on it will be clear why.

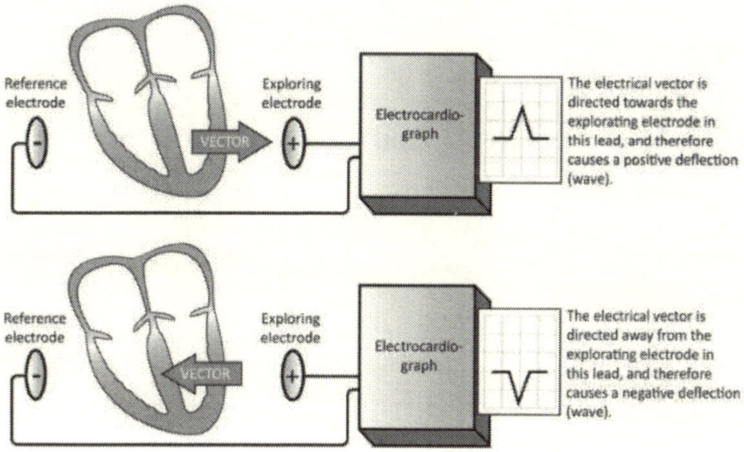

Figure 5. An ECG lead displays an ECG curve (diagram). At least two electrodes are necessary to obtain an ECG lead. One of the electrodes serves as

reference and the other serves as exploring electrode. The electrocardiograph compares the electrical potentials detected in the electrodes. If a vectors travels towards the exploring electrode, and away from the reference electrode, a positive wave is printed.

Now that the relation between electrical vectors and ECG waves has been clarified, it is time to study the main vectors of the heart and how they give rise to the classical ECG curve. Leads V1 and V5 have been selected of pedagogical reasons. V1 and V5 primarily detect vectors traveling in the horizontal plane. This is due to the placement of the exploring electrode and the reference. The exploring electrode is placed interiorly on the chest wall. The reference is slightly more complicated because it is derived by taking the average of the potentials recorded by the limb electrodes (right arm, left arm, left leg) and this yields a reference located in the chest. This will be discussed in greater detail in the next chapter but for the current discussion it is sufficient to note that the exploring electrode is located anteriorly on the chest and the reference point is located inside the chest.

Chapter 3

The ECG leads: electrodes, limb leads, chest (precordial) leads, 12-Lead ECG (EKG)

Before discussing the ECG leads and various lead systems, we need to clarify the difference between ECG leads and ECG electrodes. An **electrode** is a conductive pad which is attached to the skin and enables recording of electrical currents. An ECG **lead** is a graphical description of the electrical activity of the heart and it is created by analyzing several electrodes.

In other words, each ECG lead is computed by analyzing the electrical currents detected by several electrodes. The standard ECG – which is referred to as a 12-lead ECG since it includes 12 leads – is obtained using 10 electrodes. These 12 leads consist of two sets of ECG leads: limb leads and chest leads. The chest leads may also be referred to as *precordial leads*.

This chapter will discuss the ECG leads in detail and no prior knowledge is required. Note that the terms *unipolar leads* and *bipolar leads* are not recommended because all ECG leads are bipolar, since they compare electrical currents in two measurement points.

Electrophysiological basis of the ECG leads

Movement of charged particles generates an electrical current. In electrocardiology the charged particles are represented by intra- and extracellular ions (Na+, K+, Ca2+). These ions flow across cell membranes (so that the cell can de- and repolarize) and between cells via gap junctions (so that the depolarization can spread between the cells).

Electrical potential difference arise as the electrical impulse travels through the heart. Electric potential difference is defined as a difference in electric potential between two measurement points. In electrocardiology these measurement points are the skin electrodes. Thus, the electrical potential difference is the difference in the electrical potential detected by two (or more) electrodes.

In the previous discussion it was clarified how de- and repolarization generates electrical current. It was also explained that the electrical currents are conducted all the way to the skin, because the tissues and fluids surrounding the heart, indeed the entire human body, acts as electrical conductors. By placing electrodes on the skin it is possible to detect these electrical currents. The electrocardiograph (ECG machine) compares, amplifies and filters the electrical potential differences recorded by the electrodes and presents the results as ECG leads. Each ECG lead is presented as a diagram (sometimes called a curve).

The 12-lead ECG

Numerous ECG lead systems and constellations of leads have been tested but the standard **12-lead ECG** is still the most used and the most important lead system to master. The 12-lead ECG offers outstanding possibilities to diagnose abnormalities. Importantly, the vast majority of recommended ECG criteria (e.g criteria for acute myocardial infarction) have been derived and validated using the 12-lead ECG.

The 12-lead ECG displays, as the name implies, 12 leads which are derived by means of 10 electrodes. Three of these leads are easy to understand, since they are simply the result of comparing electrical potentials recorded by two electrodes; one electrode is exploring, while the other is a reference electrode. In the remaining 9 leads the exploring electrode is still just one electrode but the reference is obtained by combining two or three electrodes.

At any given instant during the cardiac cycle all ECG leads analyze the same electrical events but from different angles. This means that ECG leads with similar angles must display similar ECG curves (diagrams). For some purposes (e.g diagnosis of some arrhythmias) it is not always necessary to analyze all leads, as the diagnosis can often be established by examining fewer leads. On the other hand, for the purpose of diagnosis morphological changes (e.g myocardial ischemia), ability to do so increases as the number of leads increase.

The 12-lead ECG is a trade-off between sensitivity, specificity and feasibility. Obviously, having 120 leads (which has been tested in several studies on acute myocardial infarction) would improve sensitivity for many conditions, at the expense of specificity and certainly feasibility. The other extreme, using only one lead would allow for diagnosing several arrhythmias but certainly not all and more importantly it would not allow one to diagnose morphological changes in the heart. Later on it will become clear as to why multiple leads are necessary to diagnose morphological changes.

The ECG paper

The electrocardiograph presents one diagram for each lead. Voltage is presented on the vertical (Y) axis and time on the horizontal (X) axis of the diagram. The ECG paper has **small boxes** (thin lines) and **large boxes** (heavy lines). Small boxes are squares of 1 mm2 and there are 5 small boxes inside each large box. Refer to **Figure 1** below

With normal **gain** (calibration) 10 mm on the vertical axis corresponds to 1 mV. Thus, 1 mm corresponds to 0.1 mV. The amplitude (height) of a wave/deflection is measured from the maximum of the wave/deflection to the **baseline** (also called **isoelectric line**).

The ECG paper speed is generally **25 mm**/s or **50 mm/s** (10 mm/s may be used for longer recordings). All modern ECG machines can switch between these paper speeds and the choice of speed does not affect any aspect of ECG interpretation (although the waves are better delineated using 50 mm/s). Anyone aiming to become proficient in ECG interpretation must master any paper speed. The figure below (**Figure 1**) shows the differences between 50 mm/s and 25 mm/s.

This figure should be studied carefully and attention should be paid to differences on the X-axis (there are no difference with respect to the Y-axis). Both 25 mm/s and 50 mm/s will be used to present the ECG tracings in this course.

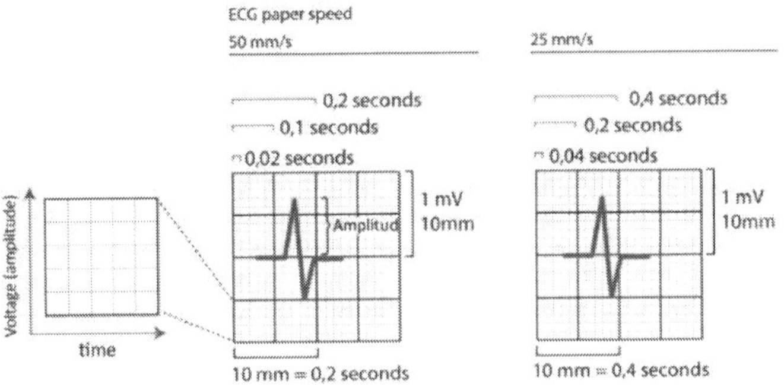

Figure 1. The ECG grid.

As evident from Figure 1:

- 1 small box (1 mm) is 0.02 seconds (20 milliseconds) at 50 mm/s.
- 1 small box (1mm) is 0.04 seconds (40 milliseconds) at 25 mm/s.
- 1 large box (5 mm) is 0.1 seconds (100 milliseconds) at 50 mm/s.
- 1 large box (5 mm) is 0.2 seconds (200 milliseconds) at 25 mm/s.

The reader should know these differences as it is often necessary to manually measure the time duration of various waves and intervals on the ECG.

Derivation of the ECG leads

Every lead represents differences in electrical potentials measured in two points in space. The simplest leads are composed using only two electrodes. The electrocardiograph defines one electrode as exploring (positive) and the other as reference (negative) electrode. In most leads, however, the reference is actually composed of a combination of two or three electrodes.

Regardless of how the exploring electrode and the reference is set up, the vectors have the same impact on the ECG curve. A vector heading towards the exploring electrode yields a positive wave/deflection and vice versa. Please refer to Figure 2 below.

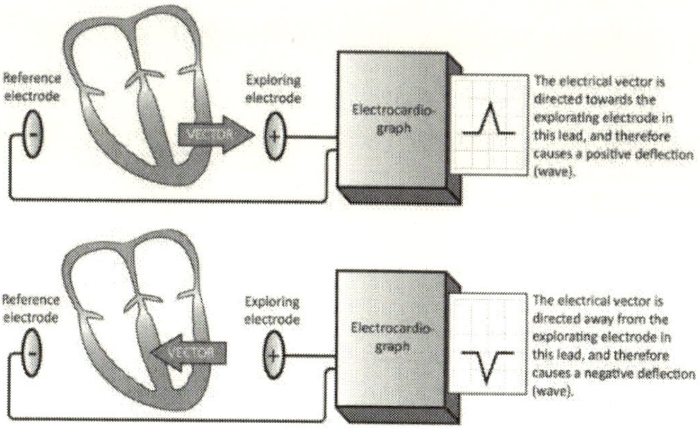

Figure 2. The electrocardiograph generates an ECG lead by comparing the electrical potential difference in two points in space. In the simplest leads these two points are two electrodes (illustrated in this figure). One electrode serves as exploring electrode (positive) and the other as the reference electrode. The electrocardiograph is constructed such that an electrical current traveling towards the exploring electrode yields a positive deflection, and vice versa.

Anatomical planes and ECG leads

The electrical activity of the heart can be observed from the horizontal plane and the frontal plane. The ability of a lead to detect vectors in a certain plane depend on how the lead is angled in relation to the plane, which in turn depend on the placement of the exploring lead and the reference point.

For pedagogical purposes, consider a lead with one electrode placed on the head and the other electrode placed on the left foot. The angle of this lead would be vertical, from the head to the foot. This lead is angled in the frontal plane and it will primarily detect vectors traveling in that plane. Refer to **Figure 3 panel A.** Now consider a lead with an electrode placed on the sternum and the other electrode placed on the back (on the same level). This lead will be angled from the back to the anterior chest wall, which is the horizontal plane. This lead will primarily record vectors traveling in that plane. A schematic illustration is provided in Figure 1 above. Refer to **Figure 3 panel B.**

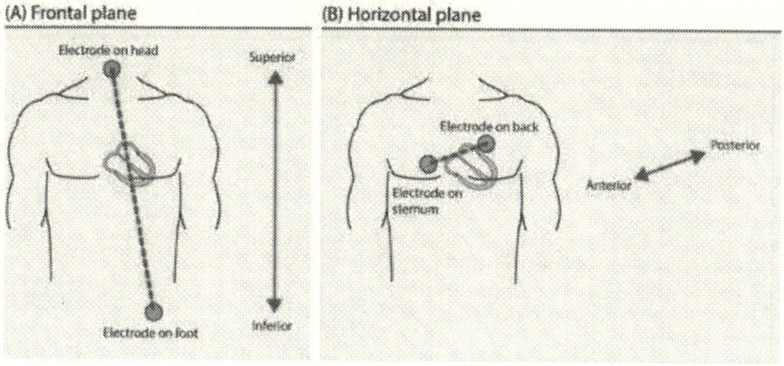

Figure 3. Schematic view of the angle of limb and chest leads.

The limb leads, of which there are six (I, II, III, aVF, aVR and aVL), have the exploring electrode and the reference point placed in the frontal plane. These leads are therefore excellent for detecting vectors traveling in the frontal plane. The chest (precordial) leads (V1, V2, V3, V4, V5 and V6) have the exploring electrodes located anteriorly on the chest wall and the reference point located inside the chest. Hence, the chest leads are excellent for detecting vectors traveling in the horizontal plane.

As noted previously only three leads, namely leads I, II and III are derived by using only two electrodes. The remaining nine leads use a reference which is composed of the average of either two or three electrodes. This will be clarified shortly.

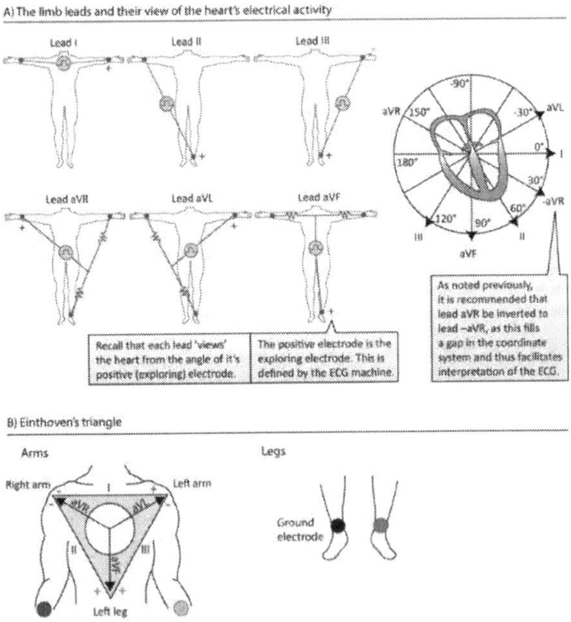

Figure 4. The organization of the limb leads. Note that the electrode on the right leg is not included in any lead, but serves as a ground wire. Leads I, II and III are Einthoven's original leads, and they can be presented with Einthoven's triangle (lower panel). Leads aVR, aVL and aVF were constructed by Goldberger; their reference point is the average of two electrodes. Lead aVR can be inverted into lead –aVR which is recommended as it may facilitate interpretation. All modern ECG machines are capable of presenting both aVR and -aVR.

Principles of the limb leads

Leads I, II, III, aVF, aVL and aVR are all derived using three electrodes, which are placed on the right arm, the left arm and the left leg. Given the electrode placements, in relation to the heart, these leads primarily detect electrical activity in the frontal plane. **Figure 4** shows how the electrodes are connected in order to obtain these six leads.

To explain derivation of the limb leads, lead I and lead aVF will be used as examples.

Considering lead I the electrode on the right arm serves as the reference, whereas the electrode on the left arm serves as the exploring electrode. This means that a vector moving from right to left should yield a positive deflection in lead I. Note that Lead I defines 0° in the frontal plane (**Figure 4**, the coordinate system in the upper panel). This also means that lead I "views" the heart from an angle of 0°. In clinical practice, it is typically expressed as if lead I "views the lateral wall of the left ventricle". The same principles apply to lead II and lead III.

In lead aVF the electrode on the left leg serves as exploring electrode and the reference is actually composed by computing the average of the arm electrodes. The average of the arm electrodes yields a reference directly north of the left leg electrode. Thus, any vector moving downwards in the chest should yield a positive wave in lead aVF. The angle by which lead aVF views the heart's electrical activity is 90° (**Figure 4**). In clinical practice, it is typically expressed as if lead aVF "views the inferior wall of the left ventricle". The same principles apply to lead aVR and lead aVL.

Lead II, aVF and III are called **inferior limb** leads, because they primarily observe the inferior wall of the left ventricle (**Figure 4, coordinate system in upper panel**). Lead aVL, I and –aVR are called **lateral limb leads**, because they primarily observe the lateral wall of the left ventricle. Note that lead aVR differs from lead –aVR (discussed below).

All six limb leads are presented in a coordinate system, which the right hand side of **Figure 4** (panel A) shows. There is 30° distance between each lead, except from the gap between lead I and lead II. To eliminate this cap, lead aVR can be inverted into lead –aVR. It turns out that this is actually meaningful, as it facilitates ECG interpretation (e.g interpretation of ischemia and electrical axis).

Whether lead aVR or –aVR is presented depend on national traditions. In the US lead aVR is used more frequently than –aVR. However, all modern ECG machines are capable of presenting both aVR and –aVR, and we recommend that –aVR be used as it facilitates ECG interpretation. In any case, the clinician can easily switch between aVR and –aVR without adjusting the ECG machine; this is done simply by turning the ECG curve upside-down.

ECG Leads I, II and III (Willem Einthoven's original leads

Leads I, II and III compare electrical potential differences between two electrodes. Lead I compares the electrode on the left arm with the electrode on the right arm, of which the former is the exploring electrode. It is said that lead I observes the heart "from the left" because its exploring electrode is placed on the left (at an angle of 0°, see **Figure 4**).

Lead II compares the left leg with the right arm, with the leg electrode being the exploring electrode. Therefore, lead II observes the heart from an angle of 60°. Lead III compares the left leg with the left arm, with the leg electrode being the exploring one. Lead III observes the heart from an angle of 120° (**Figure 4**).

Leads I, II and III are the original leads constructed by Wilhelm Einthoven. The spatial organization of these leads forms a triangle in the chest (**Einthoven's triangle**) which is presented in Figure 4, panel B.

According to **Kirchhoff's law**, the sum of all currents in a closed circuit must be zero. Since Einthoven's triangle can be viewed as a circuit, the same rule should apply to it. Thus emerges Einthoven's law:

$$\text{Lead I} + \text{Lead III} = \text{Lead II}$$

Einthoven's law.

This law implies that the sum of the potentials in lead I and lead III equals the potentials in lead II. In clinical electrocardiography this means that the amplitude of, for example, the R-wave in lead II is equal to the sum of the R-wave amplitudes in lead I and III. It follows that we need only know the information in two leads in order to calculate the exact appearance of the remaining lead. Hence, these three leads actually carry two pieces of information, observed from three angles.

ECG lead aVR, aVF and aVL (Goldberger's leads)

These leads were originally constructed by Goldberger. In these leads the exploring electrode is compared with a reference which is based on an average of the other two limb electrodes. The letter **a** stands for **augmented**, **V** for **voltage** and **R** is **right arm**, **L** is **left arm** and **F** is **foot**.

In aVR the right arm is the exploring electrode and the reference is composed by averaging the left arm and left leg. Lead aVR can be inverted into lead –aVR (which means that the exploring and reference point has switched positions), which is identical to aVR but upside-down. There are three advantages of inverting aVR into –aVR:

1. –aVR fills the gap between lead I and lead II in the coordinate system.
2. –aVR facilitates calculation of the hearts electrical axis.
3. –aVR improves diagnosis of acute ischemia/infarction (inferior and lateral ischemia/infarction).

Despite these advantages lead aVR is unfortunately still used in the United States and many other countries. Luckily, all modern ECG machines can be configured to show either aVR or –aVR. We recommend the use of –aVR but for the purpose of this book we will frequently present both leads. If only one of these leads is shown, the reader may simply turn it upside-down to get a view of the desired lead. Finally, it should be noted that very few ECG diagnoses depend on lead aVR/–aVR.

In lead aVL the left arm electrode is exploring and the lead views the heart from –30°. In lead aVF the exploring electrode is placed on the left leg, so this lead observes the heart directly from south.

Since Godlberger's leads are composed of the same electrodes as Einthoven's leads, it is not surprising that all these leads display a mathematical relation. The equations follow:

$$aVL: \quad \frac{Lead\ I - Lead\ III}{2}$$

$$-aVR: \quad \frac{Lead\ I + Lead\ II}{2}$$

$$aVF: \quad \frac{Lead\ II + Lead\ III}{2}$$

Goldberger's equations.

It follows that the ECG waves in lead aVF, at any given instance, is the average of the ECG deflection in leads II and III. Hence, leads aVR/−aVR, aVL and aVF can be calculated by using leads I, II and IIII and therefore these leads (aVF, aVR/−aVR, aVL) do not offer any new information, but instead new angles to view the same information.

Anatomical aspects of the limb leads

- **II**, **aVF** and **III**: are called **inferior** (**diaphragmal**) **limb leads** and they primarily observe the inferior aspect of the left ventricle.
- **aVL**, **I** and -**aVR**: are called **lateral limb leads**

and they primarily observe the lateral aspect of the left ventricle.

Chest leads (precordial leads)

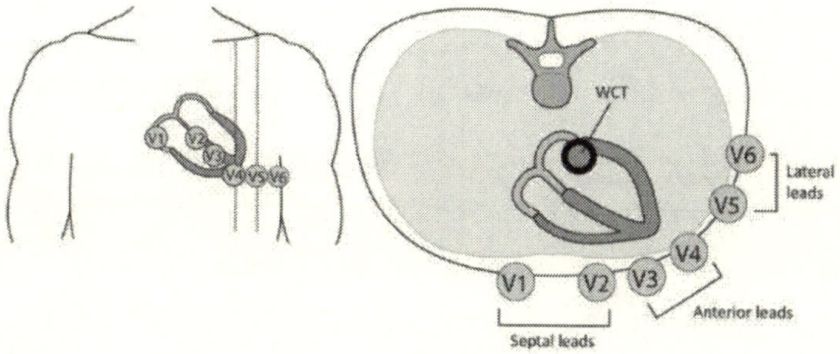

Figure 5. The chest (precordial) leads. WCT = Wilson's central terminal.

Frank Wilson and colleagues constructed the central terminal, later termed **Wilson's central terminal** (**WCT**). This terminal is a theoretical reference point located approximately in the center of thorax, or more precisely in the centre or Einthoven's triangle. WCT is computed by connecting all three limb electrodes (via electrical resistance) to one terminal.

This terminal will represent the average of the electrical potentials recorded in the limb electrodes.

Under ideal circumstances, the sum of these potentials is zero (Kirchoff’s law). WCT serves as the reference point for each of the six electrodes which are placed anteriorly on the chest wall.

The chest leads are derived by comparing the electrical potentials in WCT to the potentials recorded by each of the electrodes placed on the chest wall. There are six electrodes on the chest wall and thus six chest leads (**Figure 5**). Each chest lead offers unique information that cannot be derived mathematically from other leads. Since the exploring electrode and the reference is placed in the horizontal plane, these leads primarily observe vectors moving in that plane.

Placement of chest (precordial) electrodes

- V1: fourth intercostal space, to the right of sternum.
- V2: fourth intercostal space, to the left of sternum.
- V3: placed diagonally between V2 and V4.
- V4: between rib 5 and 6 in the midclavicular line.
- V5: placed on the same level as V4, but in the

anterior axillary line.

- V6: placed on the same level as V4 and V5, but in he midaxillary line.

Hair on the chest wall should be shaved before placement of electrodes.

Anatomical aspects of the chest (precordial) leads

- **V1-V2** ("septal leads"): primarily observes the ventricular septum, but may occasionally display ECG changes originating from the right ventricle. Note that none of the leads in the 12-lead ECG are adequate to detect vectors of the right ventricle.
- **V3-V4** ("anterior leads"): observes the anterior wall of the left ventricle.
- **V5-V6** ("anterolateral leads"): observes the lateral wall of the left ventricle.

Figure 6 shows the combined views of all leads in the 12-lead ECG.

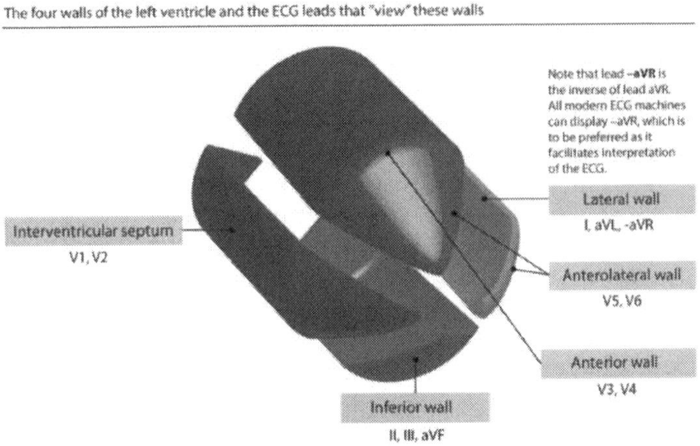

Figure 6. The 12-lead ECG records information on electrical activity of the left ventricle (and not so much of the right ventricle). As seen in the figure above the left ventricle has the shape of a bullet. The left ventricle is traditionally divided into four walls, and the figure above shows which leads that best observe electrical activity of each wall.

Presentation of ECG leads

The ECG leads may be presented chronologically (i.e I, II, III, aVL, aVR, aVL, V1 to V6) or according to their anatomical angles. Chronological order does not respect that leads aVL, I and -aVR all view the heart from a similar angle and placing them next to each other can improve diagnostics. The **Cabrera system** should be preferred. In the Cabrera system, the leads are placed in their anatomical order. The inferior limb leads (II, aVF and III) are juxtaposed, and the same goes for the lateral limb leads and the chest leads.

As mentioned earlier, inverting lead aVR into –aVR improves diagnostics additionally. All modern ECG machines can display the leads according to the Cabrera system, which should always be preferred. The ECG below shows an example of the Cabrera layout with aVR inverted into –aVR. Note the clear transition between the waveforms in neighbouring leads.

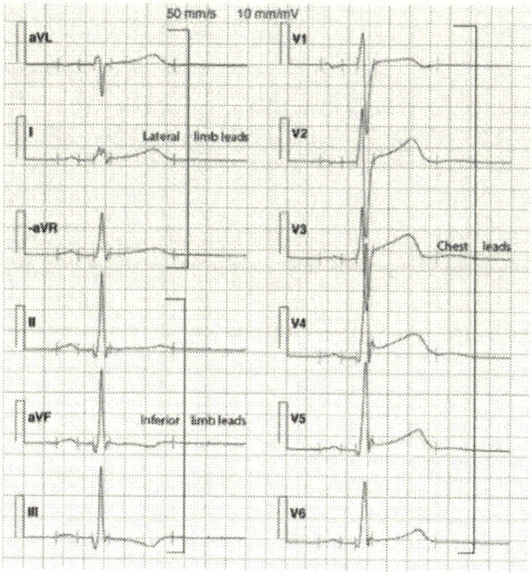

Figure 7. Presentation of the ECG leads according to the Cabrera format and aVR inverted to –aVR.

Additional (supplementary) ECG leads

There are conditions that may be missed when utilizing the 12-lead ECG. Fortunately, researchers have validated the use of additional leads to improve diagnostics of such conditions. These are now discussed.

Right ventricular ischemia/infarction: ECG leads V3R, V4R, V5R and V6R

Infarction of the right ventricle is unusual but may occur if the right coronary artery is occluded proximally. None of the standard leads in the 12-lead ECG is adequate for diagnosing right ventricular infarction. However, V1 and V2 may occasionally display ECG changes indicative of ischemia located in the right ventricle. In such scenarios, it is recommended that additional leads be placed on the right side of the chest. These leads are V3R, V4R,

V5R and V6R, which are placed on the same anatomical locations as their left sided counterparts. Refer to **Figure 8**.

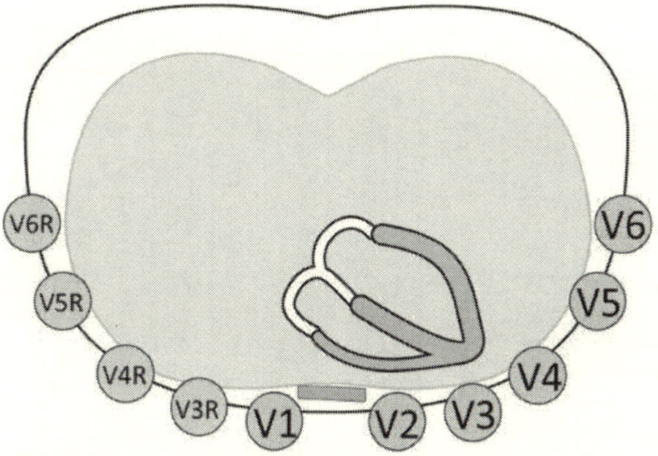

Additional leads are used when suspicion of right ventricular infarction arises. These right sided chest leads (V3R through V6R) are placed on the same locations as their left sided equivalences, but on the right side of the chest.

Figure 8. Right sided chest leads in right ventricular infarction. These leads should be connected in case there is suspicion of right ventricular infarction.

Posterolateral ischemia/infarction: ECG leads V7, V8 and V9

Considering myocardial ischemia and infarction, elevation of the ST-segment is an alarming finding as it implies that there is extensive ischemia. Ischemic ST-segment elevations are often accompanied by ST-segment depressions in ECG leads which view the ischemic vector from the opposite angle. Such ST-segment depressions are therefore termed reciprocal ST-segment depressions, because they are mirror reflections of the ST-segment elevations.

However, because the heart is rotated approximately 30° to the left in the chest (**Figure 9**), the basal parts of the lateral left ventricular wall is positioned somewhat posteriorly (which is why it is referred to as the posterolateral wall). Electrical activity emanating from this part of the left ventricle (marked with an arrow in **Figure 9**) cannot be readily detected with the standard leads, but the reciprocal changes (ST-segment depressions) are commonly seen in V1–V3.

In order to reveal the ST-segment elevations located posteriorly, one must attach the leads V7, V8 and V9 on the back of the patient.

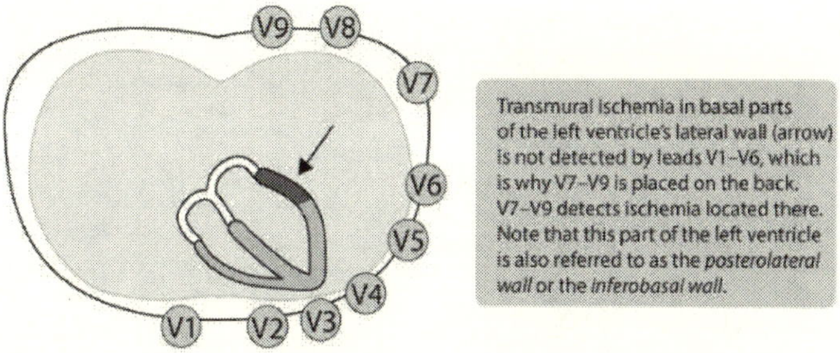

Figure 9. Posterior chest leads may reveal posterior ST-segment elevation myocardial infarction. These leads should be placed on the patient if ECG raises suspicion of posterolateral ischemia.

Alternative ECG lead systems

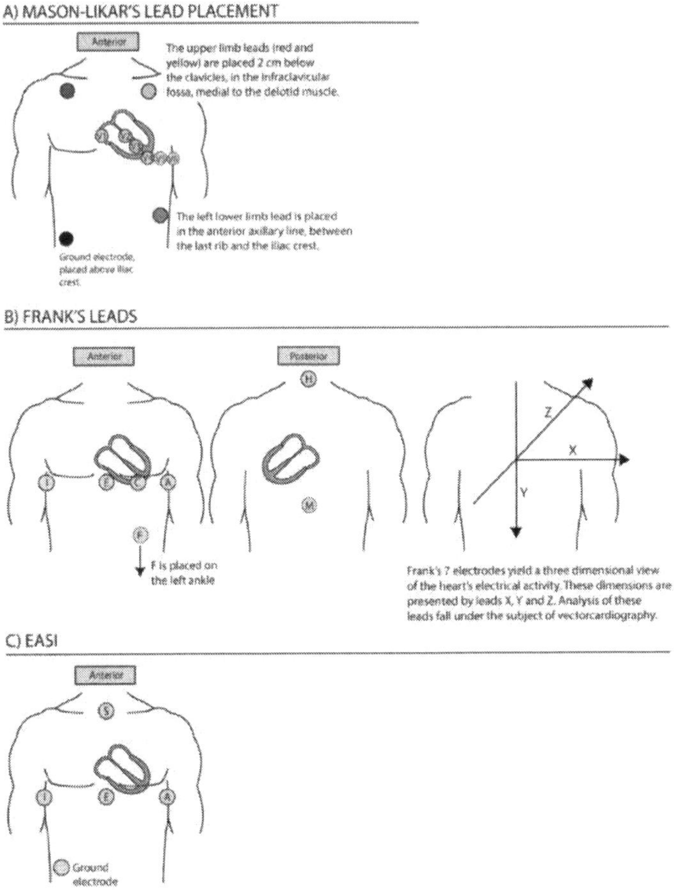

Figure 10. Alternative ECG lead systems.

The conventional placement of electrodes can be suboptimal in some situations. Electrodes placed distally on the limbs will record too much muscle disturbance during exercise stress testing; electrodes on the chest wall may be inappropriate in case of resuscitation and echocardiographic examination etc. Efforts have been made to find alternative electrode placements, as well as reducing the number of electrodes without losing information. In general, lead systems with less than 10 electrodes can still be used to compute the all standard leads in the 12-lead ECG. Such calculated ECG waveforms are very similar to the original 12-lead ECG waveforms, with some minor differences that may affect amplitudes and intervals.

As a rule of thumb, modified lead systems are fully capable of diagnosing arrhythmias but one should be cautious when using these systems to diagnose morphological conditions (e.g ischemia) that dependent on criteria for amplitudes and intervals (because the alternative electrode placement may affect these variables and cause to false positive and false negative ECG criteria). Indeed, in the setting of myocardial ischemia one millimeter may make a life-threatening difference.

Lead systems with reduced electrodes are still used

daily to detect episodes of ischemia in hospitalized patients. This is explained by the fact that when monitoring continuously – i.e when assessing ECG changes over time – the initial ECG recording is of minor importance. Instead the interest lies in the dynamics of the ECG and in that scenario the initial recording is of little interest.

Mason-Likar ECG lead system

Mason-Likar's lead system simply implies that the limb electrodes have been relocated to the trunk. This is used in all types of ECG monitoring (arrhythmias, ischemia etc). It is also used for exercise stress testing (as it avoids muscle disturbances from the limbs). As stated above, the initial recording may differ slightly (in amplitudes) so that it is not valid to diagnose ischemia on the initial tracing. For monitoring ischemia over time, however, Mason-Likar is an effective system. Refer to **Figure 10 A**.

Placement of electrodes

The left and right arm electrodes are moved to the

trunk, beneath the 2 cm beneath the clavicle, in the infraclavicular fossa (**Figure 10 A**). The left leg electrode is placed in the anterior axillary line between the iliac crest and the last rib. The right leg electrode can be placed above the iliac crest on the right side. Placement of the chest leads is not changed.

Reduced ECG lead systems

As mentioned above, it is possible to construct (mathematically) a 12-lead system with fewer than 10 electrodes. In general, mathematically derived lead systems generate ECG waveforms that are almost identical to the conventional 12-lead ECG, but only almost. The most used lead systems are Frank's and EASI.

Frank leads

Frank's system is the most common of the reduced leads system. It is generated by means of 7 electrodes (Figure 10 B). Using these leads, 3 orthogonal leads (X, Y and Z) are derived. These leads are used in vectorcardiography (VCG). Orthogonal means that the leads are perpendicular to each other. These leads offer a three-dimensional view of the cardiac vector during the cardiac cycle. The vectors are presented as loop diagrams, with separate loops for P-, QRS-, T- and the U-vector. The VCG can, however, be approximated from the 12-lead ECG, and the opposite is also true, the 12-lead ECG can be approximated from the VCG. However, the VCG has lost much ground in recent decades as it has become evident that the VCG has very low specificity for most conditions.

Placement of electrodes

The electrodes are placed horizontally in the 5th intercostal space.

- A is placed midaxillary to the left.
- C is placed between E and A.
- H is placed on the neck.
- E is placed on the sternum.
- I is placed midaxillary to the right
- M is placed on the vertebral column.
- F is placed on the left ankle.

Lead X is derived from A, C and I. Lead Y is derived from F, M and H. Lead Z is derived from A, M, I, E and C.

EASI leads

EASI provides a good approximation to the conventional 12-lead ECG. However, EASI may also generate ECG waveforms with amplitudes and durations that differ from the 12-lead ECG. This lead system is generated by using electrodes I, E and A from Frank's leads, and by adding electrode S on the manubrium. EASI also provides orthogonal information. Please refer to Figure 10.

Chapter 4

Standard display of ECG leads in the 12-lead ECG

Numerous conditions which can be diagnosed using the 12-lead ECG requires that ECG changes occur in two or more *anatomically contiguous leads*, which implies leads that are *anatomically juxtaposed*. The reason for this is simple. For example, if there is acute ischemia located in the anterior wall and there is ST segment elevation in lead V3, then there should also be ST elevation in either V2 or V4, because it is unlikely that ischemia would only be detected in one lead. Thus, leads V3 and V4 are anatomically contiguous, as are leads V2 and V3.

You have probably noticed that the chest leads (V1 through V6) are displayed on the ECG paper in their anatomically contiguous order from right anterior (V1) to left lateral (V6), but regrettably the limb leads are not. Instead, the limb leads are displayed in two groups of three: leads I, II and III and leads aVR, aVL and aVF. **Figure 1** shows the traditional presentation of the 12-lead ECG. This presentation format is the standard in the United States, United Kingdom, most parts of Europe, South America, Asia and Africa.

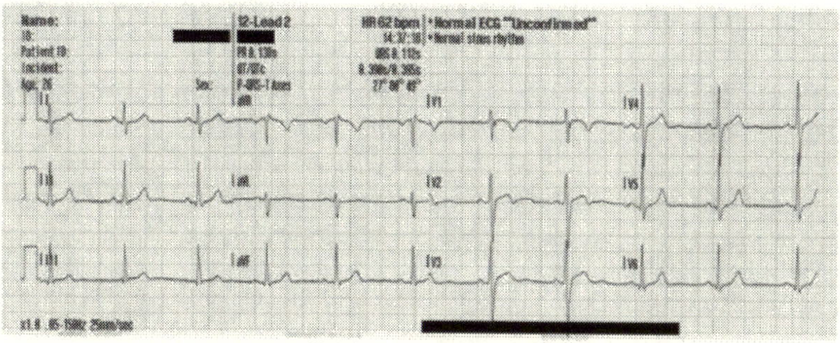

Figure 1. Traditional presentation of the leads in the 12-lead ECG.

The Cabrera format of the 12-lead ECG

As evident in **Figure 1**, the traditional presentation of the ECG leads is not particularly helpful. Presentation of leads I, II, III, aVR, aVL and aVF actually reflects their historical development. Leads I, II and III were developed by Einthoven and leads aVR, aVL and aVF were developed by Goldberger. This presentation makes ECG interpretation more difficult and time consuming, because the reader must go back and forth between the leads on the paper.

It would be more efficient to present the limb leads in their anatomically contiguous manner; that is, from left superior-basal to right inferior. In other word, the following order: aVL, I, −aVR (i.e., lead aVR with reversed polarity), II, aVF, and III. Note that lead –aVR exists at 30° in the frontal plane, according to **Figure 2**.

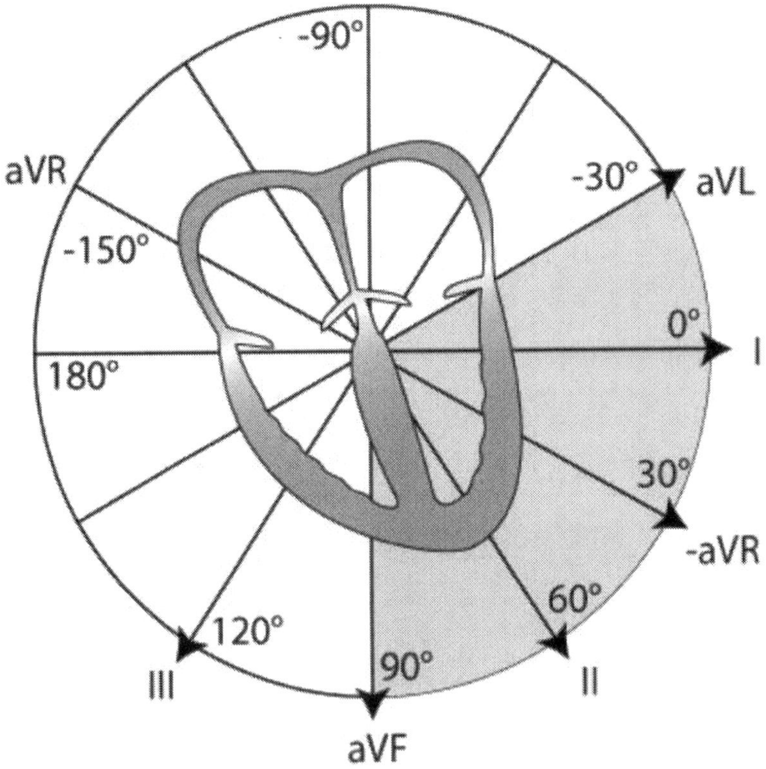

Figure 2. The coordinate system presenting the limb leads in the frontal plane.

This format of displaying the ECG leads is referred to as the **Cabrera format** and it has been the existing standard in Sweden for over 30 years. Let's have a look at the standard 12-lead ECG with the Cabrera format (**Figure 3**):

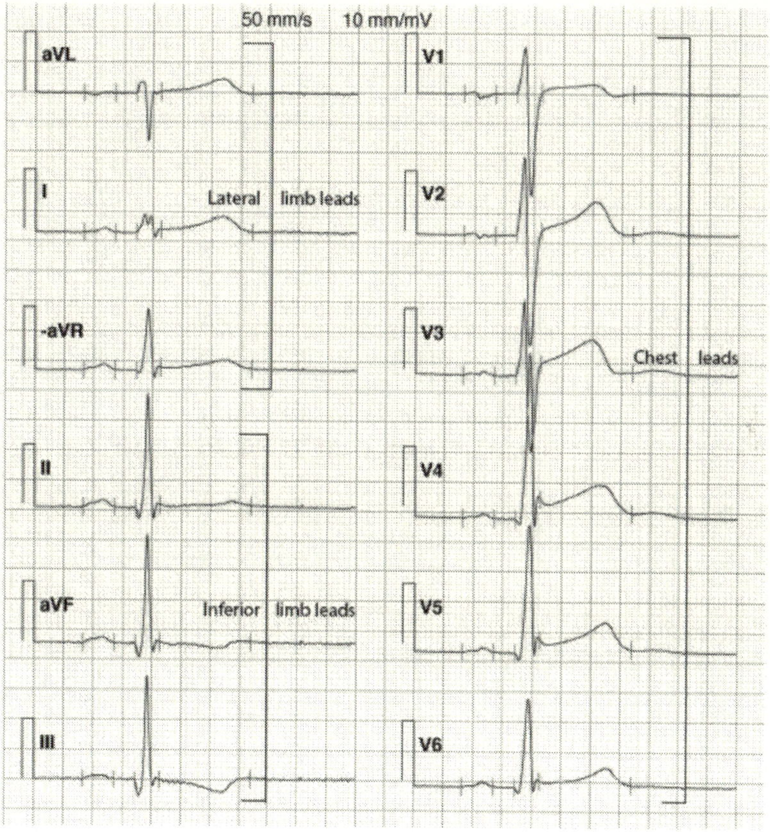

Figure 3. The Cabrera format and inverted aVR.

It is clear that the reader will find it much easier to study the inferior and lateral wall using the Cabrera display. As evident in Figure 3, if leads I, II and III would have been displayed next to each other, the T-wave inversion in lead III would not be consistent with the upright T-waves in leads I and II. However, placing lead III next to aVF makes more sense, because aVF also displays a negative T-wave and the reader will be able to spot that directly!

The American College of Cardiology (ACC), The European Society for Cardiology (ESC) and the American Heart Association (AHA) has recommended that there should be universal adoption of the Cabrera format. This recommendation, [1] was issued 16 years ago and fortunately all modern ECG machines can switch to the Cabrera format (including –aVR). We encourage the use of the Cabrera format in order to facilitate ECG interpretation.

Lead –aVR: the inverted lead aVR

As evident in **Figure 2** there is 30° distance between

each limb lead, except from the gap between lead I and lead II. To eliminate this gap, lead aVR can be inverted into lead –aVR. To obtain lead –aVR, the exploring and the reference points must switch positions, so that lead –aVR is actually equal to aVR upside-down. It turns out that the use of lead –aVR is actually meaningful, as it facilitates ECG interpretation (e.g interpretation of myocardial ischemia and electrical axis).

All modern ECG machines can present either aVR or -aVR; we recommend that –aVR be used as it facilitates ECG interpretation. In any case, the reader can easily switch between aVR and –aVR without adjusting the ECG machine; by simply turning the ECG curve upside-down.

Advantages of using lead –aVR instead of aVR

There are three advantages of inverting aVR into -aVR:

1. –aVR fills the gap between lead I and lead II in the coordinate system.

2. –aVR facilitates calculation of the hearts electrical axis.
3. –aVR improves diagnosis of acute ischemia/infarction (inferior and lateral ischemia/infarction).

Chapter 5

ECG Interpretation: definitions, criteria, and characteristics of the normal ECG (EKG) waves, intervals, durations & rhythm

At the heart of ECG interpretation lies the ability to determine whether the ECG waves and intervals are normal. This chapter will focus on the ECG waves in terms of morphology (appearance), durations and intervals. A rather extensive discussion is provided in order to give the reader firm knowledge of normal findings, normal variants (i.e less common variants of what is considered normal) and pathological variants. Thus, in this chapter, you will learn the physiological basis of all ECG waves and how to determine whether the ECG is normal or abnormal.

Overview of the normal electrocardiogram (ECG)

ECG interpretation includes an assessment of the morphology (appearance) of the waves and intervals on the ECG curve. Therefore, ECG interpretation requires a structured assessment of the waves and intervals. Before discussing each component in detail, a brief overview of the waves and intervals is given.

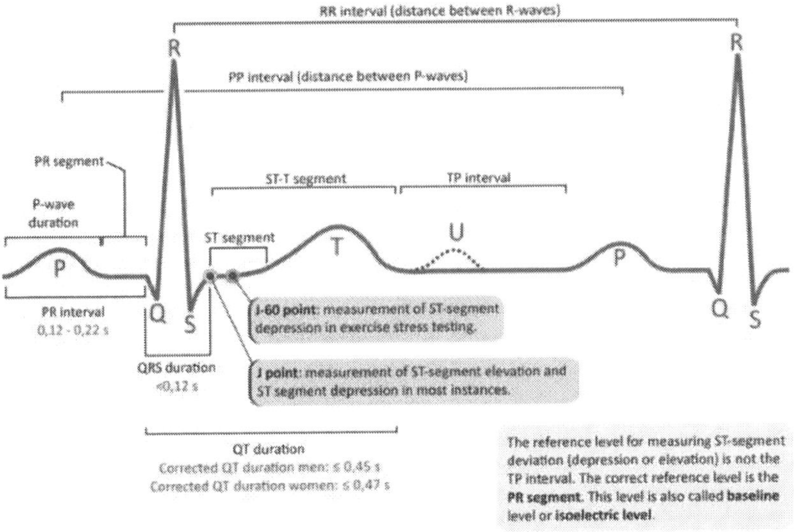

Figure 1. The classical ECG curve with its most common waveforms. Important intervals and points of measurement are depicted. ECG interpretation requires knowledge of these waves and intervals.

The P-wave, PR interval and PR segment

ECG interpretation traditionally starts with an assessment of the P-wave. The **P-wave** reflects atrial depolarization (activation). The **PR interval** is the distance between the onset of the P-wave to the onset of the QRS complex. The PR interval is assessed in order to determine whether impulse conduction from the atria to the ventricles is normal. The flat line between the end of the P-wave and the onset of the QRS complex is called the **PR segment** and it reflects the slow impulse conduction through the atrioventricular node. The PR segment serves as the baseline (also referred to as **reference line** or **isoelectric line**) of the ECG curve. The amplitude of any deflection/wave is measured by using the PR segment as the baseline. Refer to **Figure 1**.

The QRS complex

The **QRS complex** represents the depolarization (activation) of the ventricles. It is always referred to as the "QRS complex" although it may not always display all three waves. Since the electrical vector generated by the left ventricle is many times larger than the vector generated by the right ventricle, the QRS complex is actually a reflection of left ventricular depolarization. **QRS duration** is the time interval from the onset to the end of the QRS complex.

A short QRS complex is desirable as it proves that the

ventricles are depolarized rapidly, which in turn implies that the conduction system functions properly. Wide (also referred to as broad) QRS complexes indicate that ventricular depolarization is slow, which may be due to dysfunction in the conduction system.

The J point and the ST segment

The **ST segment** corresponds to the plateau phase (phase 2) of the action potential. The ST segment must always be studied carefully since it is altered in a wide range of conditions. Many of these conditions cause rather characteristic ST segment changes. The ST segment is of particular interest in the setting of acute myocardial ischemia because ischemia causes deviation of the ST segment (**ST segment deviation**). There are two types of ST segment deviations. **ST segment depression** implies that the ST segment is displaced, such that it is below the level of the PR segment. **ST segment elevation** implies that the ST segment is displaced, such that it is above the level of the PR segment.

The magnitude of depression/elevation is measured

as the height difference (in millimeters) between the **J point** and the PR segment. The J point is the point where the ST segment starts. If the baseline (PR segment) is difficult to discern, the **TP interval** may be used as the reference level.

The T-wave

The T-wave reflects the rapid repolarization of contractile cells (phase 3) and T-wave changes occur in a wide range of conditions. T-wave changes are frequently misunderstood in clinical practice, which the discussion below will attempt to cure. The transition from the ST segment to the T-wave should be smooth (and not abrupt). The normal T-wave is slightly asymmetric, with a steeper downward slope.

The U-wave

The U-wave is seen occasionally. It is a positive wave occurring after the T-wave. Its amplitude is generally one-fourth of the T-wave's amplitude. The U-wave is most frequently seen in leads V2–V4. Individuals with prominent T-waves, as well as those with slow heart rates, display U-waves more often. The genesis of the U-wave remains elusive.

QT duration and QTc duration

QT duration reflects the total duration of ventricular depolarization and repolarization. It is measured from the onset of the QRS complex to the end of the T-wave. The QT duration is inversely related to heart rate; i.e the QT interval increases at slower heart rates and decreases at higher heart rates. Therefore to determine whether the QT interval is within normal limits, it is necessary to adjust for the heart rate. The heart rate adjusted QT interval is referred to as the **corrected QT interval** (QTc interval). A long QTc interval increases the risk of ventricular arrhythmias.

Now follows the detailed discussion of each ECG of these components.

The P-wave

ECG interpretation usually starts with an assessment of the P-wave. The P-wave is a small, positive and smooth wave. It is small because the atria make a relatively small muscle mass. If the rhythm is sinus rhythm (i.e under normal circumstances) the P-wave vector is directed downwards and to the left in the frontal plane and this yield a positive P-wave in lead II (**Figure 2**, right-hand side). The P-wave is always positive in lead II during sinus rhythm. This is rather easy to understand because lead II is angled alongside the P-wave vector, and the exploring electrode is located in front of the P-wave vector (**Figure 2**, right-hand side).

The P-wave vector is slightly curved in the horizontal plane. It is initially directed forward but then turns left to activate the left atrium (**Figure 2**, left-hand side). Lead V1 might therefore display a **biphasic** (**diphasic**) **P-wave**, meaning that the greater portion of the P-wave is positive but the terminal portion is slightly negative (the vector generated by left atrial activation heads away from V1). Occasionally, the negative deflection is also seen in lead V2. lead V5 only notes vectors heading towards the exploring electrode (albeit with somewhat varying angles) and therefore displays a positive P-wave throughout.

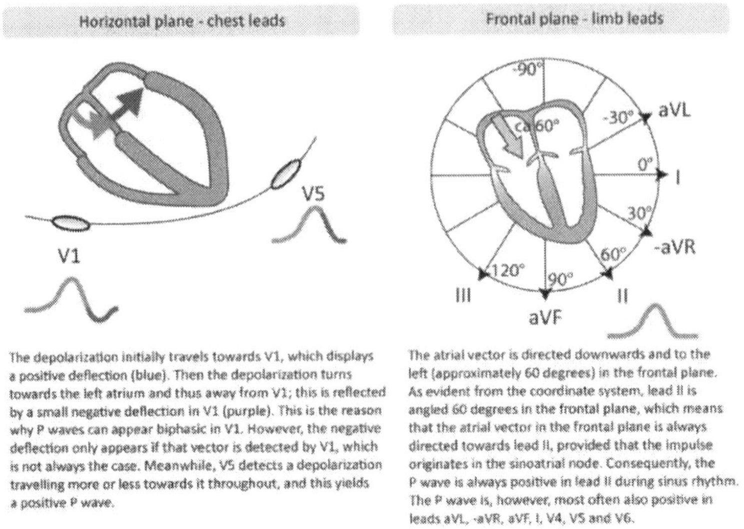

Figure 2. P-wave morphology in chest and limb leads.

Figure 2 (above) does not show that the P-wave in lead II might actually be slightly asymmetric by having two humps. This is often (but not always) seen on ordinary ECG tracings and it is explained by the fact that the atria are depolarized sequentially, with the right atrium being depolarized before the left atrium. The first half of the P-wave is therefore a reflection of right atrial depolarization and the second half is a reflection of left atrial depolarization. This is shown in Figure 3 (upper panel). Recall that the P-wave in V1 is often biphasic, which is also shown in

Figure 3.

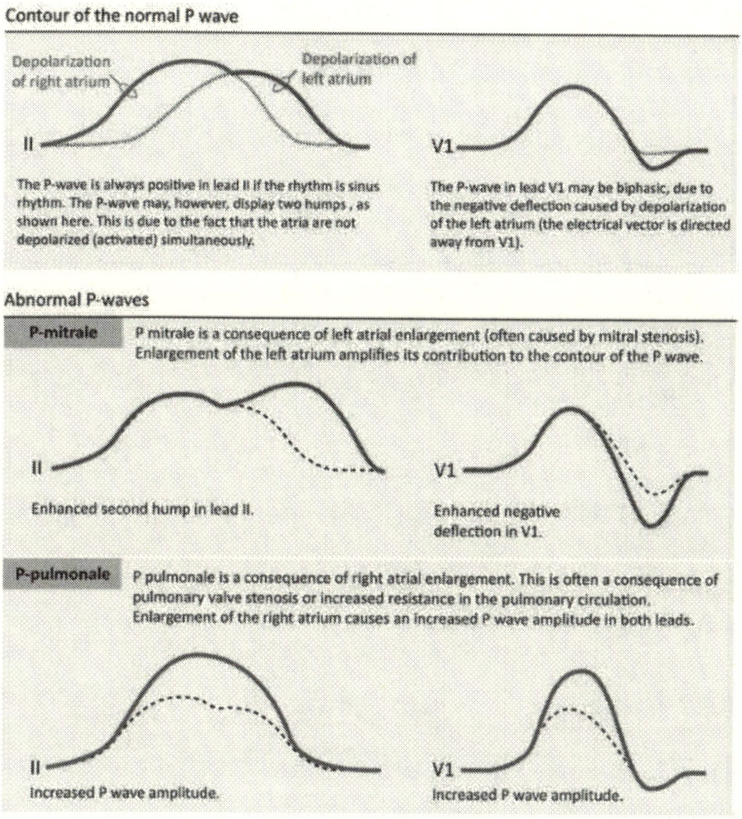

Figure 3. The contour of the normal and abnormal P-wave (P pulmonale and P mitrale).

If an atria becomes enlarged (typically as a compensatory mechanism) its contribution to the P-wave will be enhanced. Enlargement of the left and right atria causes typical P-wave changes in lead II and lead V1 (**Figure 3**).

Enlargement of the right atrium is commonly a consequence of increased resistance to empty blood into the right ventricle. This may be due to pulmonary valve stenosis, increased pulmonary artery pressure etc. The right atrium must then enlarge (hypertrophy) in order to manage to pump blood into the right ventricle. Right atrial enlargement (hypertrophy) leads to stronger electrical currents and thus enhancement of the contribution of the right atrium to the P-wave. The P-wave will display higher amplitude in lead II and lead V1. Such a P-wave is called **P pulmonale** because pulmonary disease is the most common cause (Figure 3, P-pulmonale).

If the left atrium encounters increased resistance (e.g due to mitral valve stenosis) it becomes enlarged (hypertrophy) which amplifies its contribution to the P-wave. The second hump in lead II becomes larger and the negative deflection in V1 becomes deeper. This is called **P mitrale**, because mitral valve disease is a common cause (**Figure 25**, **P-mitrale**).

If the atria are depolarized by impulses generated by cells outside of the sinoatrial node (i.e by an ectopic focus), the morphology of the P-wave may differ from the P-waves in sinus rhythm. If the ectopic focus is located close to the sinoatrial node, the P-wave will have a morphology similar to the P-wave in sinus rhythm. However, an ectopic focus may be located anywhere. If it is located near the atrioventricular node, the activation of the atria will proceed in the opposite direction, which produces an **inverted (retrograde) P-wave.**

P-wave checklist

- The P-wave is always positive in lead II during sinus rhythm.
- The P-wave is virtually always positive in leads aVL, aVF, –aVR, I, V4, V5 and V6. It is negative in lead aVR.
- The P-wave is frequently biphasic in V1 (occasionally in V2). The negative deflection is normally <1 mm.
- P-wave duration should be ≤0,12 seconds.

- P-wave amplitude should be <2,5 mm in the limb leads.
- P-pulmonale implies that the P-wave has an abnormally high amplitude in lead II (and in other leads in general).
- P-mitrale implies that the second hump of the P-wave in lead II and the negative deflection of the P-wave in lead V1 are both enhanced.

PR interval and PR segment

The PR interval starts at the onset of the P-wave and ends at the onset of the QRS complex (**Figure 1**). It reflects the time interval from the start of atrial depolarization to start of ventricular depolarization. The PR interval is assessed in order to determine whether impulse conduction from the atria to the ventricles is normal in terms of speed. The PR interval must not be too long nor too short. A normal PR interval ranges between 0.12 seconds to 0.22seconds.

The flat line between the end of the P-wave and the onset of the QRS complex is called the **PR segment** and it reflects the slow impulse conduction through the atrioventricular node. The PR segment serves as the baseline (also referred to as **reference line** or **isoelectric line**) of the ECG curve. The amplitude of any deflection/wave is measured by using the PR segment as the baseline.

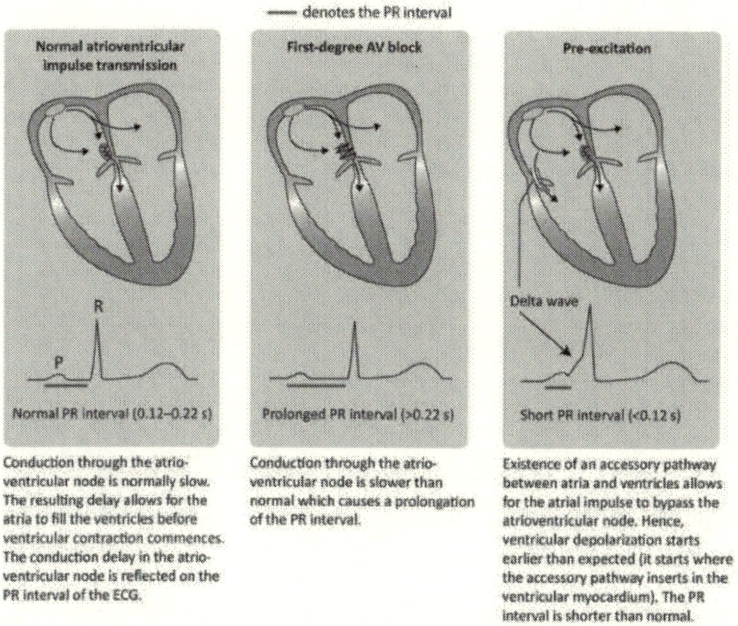

Figure 4. Impulse transmission from the atria to the ventricles. The PR interval reflects whether the impulse transmission through the AV-node is normal (first panel), abnormally slow (second panel) or bypassed (third panel).

Numerous conditions can diminish the capacity of the atrioventricular node to conduct the atrial impulse to the ventricles. As the conduction diminishes, the PR interval becomes longer. When the PR interval exceeds 0.22 seconds, **first-degree AV-block** is manifest. The term block is somewhat misleading since it is actually a matter of abnormal delay and not a block per se. The most common cause of first-degree AV-block is degenerative (age-related) fibrosis in the conduction system.

Myocardial ischemia/infarction and medications (e.g beta-blockers) may also cause first-degree AV-block. Note that the upper reference limit (0.22 seconds) should be related to the age of the patient; 0.20 seconds is more suitable for young adults because they have faster impulse conduction. Refer to **Figure 4** (second panel). AV-blocks are discussed in detail later.

The atrioventricular (AV) node is normally the only connection between the atria and the ventricles. The atria and the ventricles are electrically isolated from each other by the fibrous rings (anulus fibrosus). However, it is not rare to have an additional - accessory - pathway between the atria and the ventricles. Such an accessory pathway is an embryological remnant which may be located almost anywhere between the atria and the ventricles. It enables the atrial impulse to pass directly to the ventricles and start ventricular depolarization prematurely. If the atrial impulse uses an accessory pathway, the impulse delay in the atrioventricular node is bypassed and therefore the PR interval becomes shortened (PR interval <0.12 seconds).

The condition is referred to as **pre-excitation** because the ventricles are excited prematurely. This is illustrated in **Figure 4** (third panel). As seen in **Figure 4** (third panel) the initial depolarization of the ventricles (starting where the accessory pathway inserts into the ventricular myocardium) is slow because the impulse will not spread via the normal His-Purkinje pathway. The slow initial depolarization is seen as a **delta wave** on the ECG (**Figure 4**, third panel). However, apart from the delta wave, the R-wave will appear normal because ventricular depolarization will be executed normally as soon as the atrioventricular node delivers the impulse to the His-Purkinje system.

PR interval checklist

- Normal PR interval: 0,12–0,22 seconds. Upper reference limit is 0,20 seconds in young adults.
- A prolonged PR interval (>0.22 s) is consistent with first-degree AV-block.
- A shortened PR interval (<0,12 s) indicates pre-excitation (presence of an accessory pathway). This is associated with a delta wave.

The QRS complex (ventricular complex)

A complete QRS complex consists of a Q-, R- and S-wave. However, all three waves may not be visible and there is always variation between the leads. Some leads may display all waves, whereas others might only display one of the waves. Regardless of which waves are visible, the wave(s) that reflect ventricular depolarization is always referred to as the *QRS complex.*

Naming of the waves in the QRS complex:

Naming of the waves in the QRS complex is easy but frequently misunderstood. The following rules apply when naming the waves:

- A deflection is only referred to as a wave if it passes the baseline.
- If the first wave is negative then it is referred to as Q-wave. If the first wave is not negative, then the QRS complex does not possess a Q-wave, regardless of the appearance of the QRS complex.
- All positive waves are referred to as R-waves. The first positive wave is simply an "R-wave" (R). The second positive wave is called "R-prime wave" (R'). If a third positive wave occurs (rare) it is referred to as "R-bis wave" (R").
- Any negative wave occurring after a positive wave is an S-wave.
- Large waves are referred to by their capital letters (Q, R, S), and small waves are referred to

by their lower-case letters (q, r, s).

Figure 5 shows examples of the naming of the QRS-complex.

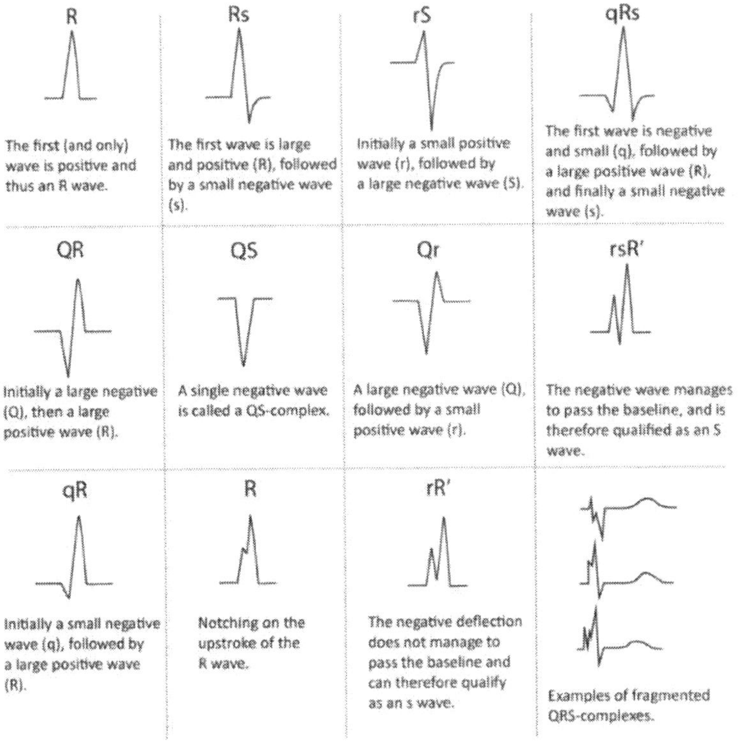

Figure 5. Naming of the QRS complex.

Net direction of the QRS complex

The QRS complex can be classified as net positive or net negative, referring to its net direction. The QRS complex is net positive if the sum of the positive areas (above baseline) exceeds that of the negative areas (below baseline). Refer to **Figure 6**, panel A. These calculations are approximated simply by eyeballing. Panel **B** in **Figure 6** shows a net negative QRS complex because the negative areas are greater than the positive area.

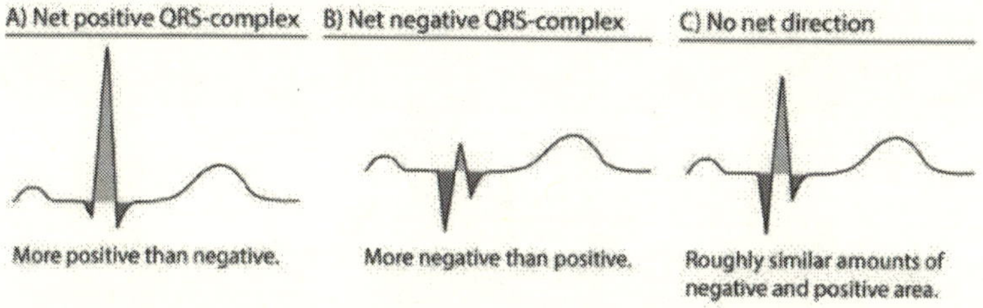

Figure 6. Approximations of the net direction of the QRS-complex. The positive areas are yellow and the negative areas are green.

Electrical vectors that engender the QRS complex

Depolarization of the ventricles generates three large vectors, which explains why the QRS complex is composed of three waves. It is fundamental to understand the genesis of these waves and although it has been discussed previously a brief rehearsal is warranted. **Figure 7** illustrates the vectors in the horizontal plane. Study Figure 7 carefully, as it illustrates how the P-wave and QRS complex are generated by the electrical vectors.

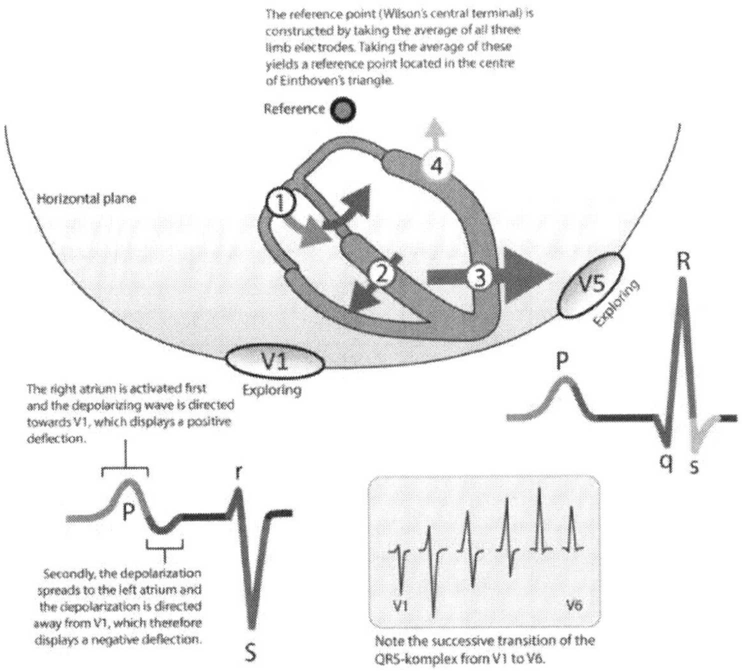

Figure 7. The heart's main electrical vectors seen from the horizontal plane. V1 and V5 are exploring electrodes and the reference is composed of the average of the electrodes placed on the limbs (this reference is called Wilson's central terminal). Inspired by MacFarlane et al (Springer, Comprehensive

Electrocardiology, 2010).

Note that the first vector in Figure 7 is not discussed here as it belongs to atrial activity.

The second vector: the ventricular (interventricular) septum

The ventricular septum receives Purkinje fibers from the left bundle branch and therefore depolarization proceeds from its left side towards its right side. The vector is directed forward and to the right. The ventricular septum is relatively small, which is why V1 displays a small positive wave (r-wave) and V5 displays a small negative wave (q-wave). Thus, it is the same electrical vector that results in an r-wave in V1 and q-wave in V5.

The third vector: the ventricular free wall

The vectors resulting from activation of the ventricular free walls is directed to the left and downwards (**Figure 7**). The explanation for this is as follows:

- **The vector resulting from activation of the right ventricle does not come to expression**, because it is drowned by the many times larger vector generated by the left ventricle. Thus, the vector during activation of the ventricular free walls is actually the vector generated by the left ventricle.
- **Activation of the ventricular free wall proceeds from the endocardium to the epicardium**. This is because the Purkinje fibers run through the endocardium, where they deliver the action potential to contractile cells. The subsequent spread of the action potential occurs from one contractile cell to another, starting in the endocardium and heading towards the epicardium.

As evident from **Figure 7**, the vector of the ventricular free wall is directed to the left (and downwards). Lead V5 detects a very large vector heading towards it and therefore displays a large R-wave. Lead V1 records the opposite and therefore displays a large negative wave called S-wave.

The fourth vector: basal parts of the ventricles

The final vector stems from activation of the basal parts of the ventricles. The vector is directed backward and upwards. It heads away from V5 which records a negative wave (s-wave). Lead V1 does not detect this vector.

Implications and causes of wide (broad) QRS complex

Prolongation of QRS duration implies that ventricular depolarization is slower than normal. The QRS duration is generally <0,10 seconds but must be <0,12 seconds. If QRS duration is ≥ 0,12 seconds (120 milliseconds) then the QRS complex is abnormally wide (broad). This is very common and a significant finding. The reason for wide QRS complexes must always be clarified. Clinicians often perceive this as a difficult task despite the fact that the list of differential diagnoses is rather short. The following causes of wide QRS complexes must be familiar to all clinicians:

- **Bundle branch block**: The left and the right bundle branch consists of Purkinje fibers which spread out into the ventricular myocardium. The Purkinje network enables fast impulse conduction so that the action potential can be delivered to the whole myocardium at the same time (approximately). Bundle branch block occurs if a bundle branch is dysfunctional and unable to transmit the impulse. The ventricle whose bundle is blocked will have to wait for electrical impulses to spread from the other ventricle. Because the spread of the impulse from the other ventricle will take place partly or entirely outside of the conduction system, it will be slow and therefore the QRS duration is prolonged.

- **Hyperkalemia**: Hyperkalemia causes slow impulse transmission (in all myocardial and conduction cells) and prolongation of the QRS duration.
- **Drugs**: class I antiarrhythmic drugs, tricyclic antidepressants, and other medications can cause widening of the QRS complex.
- **Ventricular rhythm, ventricular ectopy, and pacemaker with ventricular stimulation:**

- Spontaneous action potentials discharged within the ventricles may depolarize the ventricles. The cell/structure which discharges the action potential is referred to as an ectopic focus. Such a focus may fire single or multiple impulses (either consecutively or intermittently). *A single impulse gives rise to a premature ventricular beat, whereas multiple impulses may establish a ventricular rhythm, or even ventricular tachycardia*. In all these instances the QRS complex will be broad because the depolarizing impulse arises and spreads outside of the normal conduction system.
- External (artificial) pacemakers have an electrode inserted in the right ventricular apex. Electrical stimulation in the right ventricular apex will give rise to an action potential propagating from there, i.e partly or entirely outside of the conduction system (which will cause wide QRS complexes).

- **Pre-excitation (Wolff-Parkinson-White syndrome):** Pre-excitation implies the existence of an accessory pathway (in addition to the atrioventricular node) between the atria and the ventricles. Such pathways virtually always insert into the ventricular myocardium, from where the action potential spreads. Again, the spread takes place outside of the conduction system which is slow and causes widening of the QRS complex.
- **Aberrant ventricular conduction (aberrancy):** Aberrant conduction is actually a bundle branch block which occurs when the length of the cardiac cycle is rapidly changed, particularly at high heart rates. The bundle branches (particularly the right bundle branch) may occasionally fail to adapt their repolarization period to the length of the cardiac cycle (which they also do).

Figure 8 (below) shows examples of normal and abnormally wide QRS complexes at 25 mm/s and 50 mm/s paper speed.

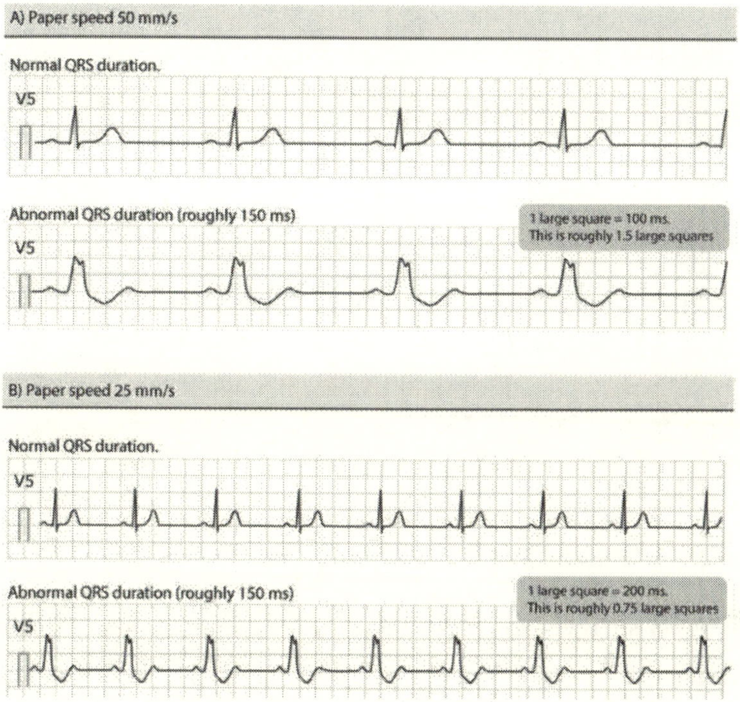

Figure 8. Normal and abnormal QRS durations at different paper speeds.

Amplitude of the QRS complex

A QRS complex with large amplitudes may be explained by ventricular hypertrophy or enlargement (or a combination of both). The electrical currents generated by the ventricular myocardium are proportional to the ventricular muscle mass. Hypertrophy means that there are more muscle and hence larger electrical potentials generated. However, the distance between the heart and the electrodes may have a significant impact on the amplitudes of the QRS complex. For example, slender individuals generally have a shorter distance between the heart and the electrodes, as compared with obese individuals. Therefore, the slender individual may present with much larger QRS amplitudes. Similarly, a person with chronic obstructive pulmonary disease (COPD) often displays diminished QRS amplitudes due to hyperinflation of thorax (increased distance to electrodes). Low amplitudes may also be caused by hypothyreosis. In the setting of circulatory collapse, low amplitudes should raise suspicion of cardiac tamponade.

R-wave amplitude

It is important to assess the amplitude of the R-waves. High amplitudes may be due to ventricular enlargement or hypertrophy. To determine whether the amplitudes are enlarged, the following references are at hand:

- R-wave should be < 26 mm in V5 and V6.
- R-wave amplitude in V5 + S-wave amplitude in V1 should be <35 mm.
- R-wave amplitude in V6 + S-wave amplitude in V1 should be <35 mm.
- R-wave amplitude in aVL should be ≤ 12 mm.
- R-wave amplitude in leads I, II and III should all be ≤ 20 mm.
- If R-wave in V1 is larger than S-wave in V1, the R-wave should be <5 mm.

(1 mm corresponds to 0.1 mV on standard ECG grid).

R-wave peak time

R-wave peak time (Figure 9) is the interval from the beginning of the QRS-complex to the apex of the R-wave. This interval reflects the time elapsed for the depolarization to spread from the endocardium to the epicardium. R-wave peak time is prolonged in hypertrophy and conduction disturbances.

Normal values for R-wave peak time follow:

- Leads V1-V2 (right ventricle) <0,035 seconds
- Leads V5-V6 (left ventricle) <0,045 seconds

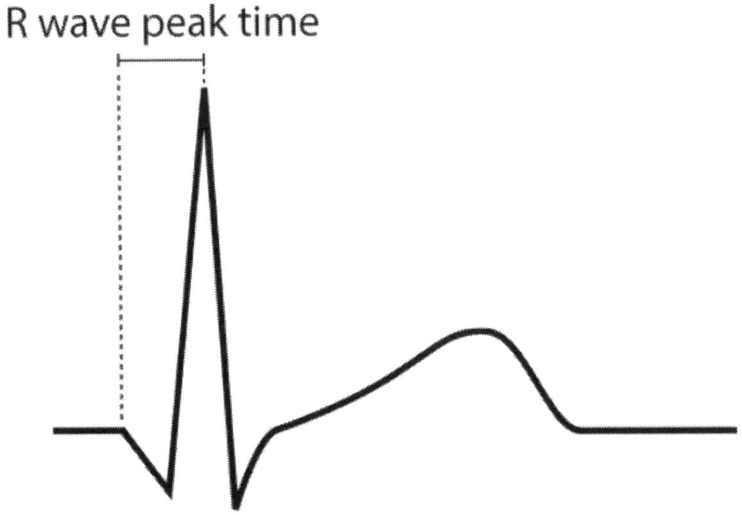

Figure 9. R-wave peak time is defined as the time interval between onset of the QRS complex to the apex of the R-wave.

R-wave progression

R-wave progression is assessed in the chest (precordial) leads. Normal R-wave progression implies that the R-wave gradually increases in amplitude from V1 to V5 and then diminishes in amplitude from V5 to

V6 (**Figure 10**, left-hand side). The S-wave undergoes the opposite development. Abnormal R-wave progression is a common finding which may be explained by any of the following conditions:

- **Myocardial infarction**: necrotic myocardium does not generate electrical potentials and therefore there is a loss of R-wave amplitude in the ECG leads reflecting the necrotic area (**Figure 10**, right-hand side).
- **Cardiomyopathy** may cause either loss or gain of R-wave amplitude, depending on the type of cardiomyopathy. Amplitudes may be increased in hypertrophic cardiomyopathy, whereas they are typically diminished in late stages of dilated cardiomyopathy.
- **Right and left ventricular hypertrophy** also amplifies the R-wave amplitude. Left ventricular hypertrophy causes increased R-wave amplitudes in V4–V6 and deeper S-waves in V1–V3. Right ventricular hypertrophy causes large R-waves in V1–V3 and smaller R-waves in V4–V6.

- **Pre-excitation, bundle branch block and chronic obstructive pulmonary disease (COPD)** may also affect R-wave progression. These conditions are discussed in detail later on.

Note that the R-wave is occasionally missing in V1 (may be due to misplacement of the electrode). This is considered a normal finding provided that an R-wave is seen in V2.

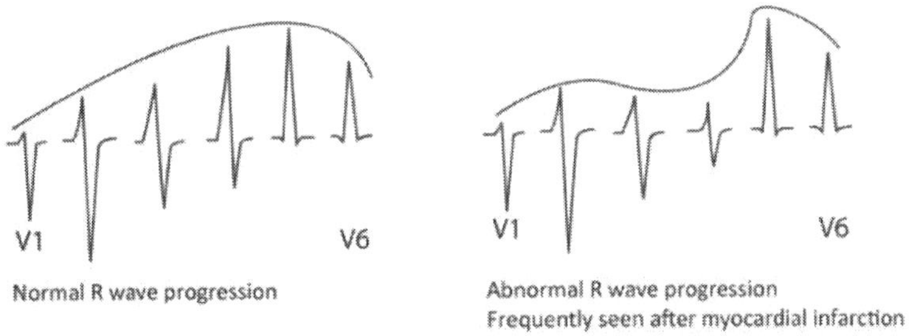

Figure 10. Normal and abnormal R-wave progression.

Dominant R-wave in V1/V2

As seen in **Figure 10** (left-hand side) the R-wave in V1–V2 is considerably smaller than the S-wave in V1–V2. Dominant R-wave in V1/V2 implies that the R-wave is larger than the S-wave, and this may be pathological. If the R-wave is larger than the S-wave, the R-wave should be <5 mm, otherwise the R-wave is abnormally large. This may be explained by right bundle branch block, right ventricular hypertrophy, hypertrophic cardiomyopathy, posterolateral ischemia/infarction (if the patient experiences chest pain), pre-excitation, dextrocardia or misplacement of chest electrodes.

The Q-wave

It is crucial to differentiate normal from pathological Q-waves, particularly because pathological Q-waves are rather firm evidence of previous myocardial infarction. However, there are numerous other causes of Q-waves, both normal and pathological and it is important to differentiate these.

The amplitude (depth) and the duration (width) of the Q-wave dictate whether it is abnormal or not. Pathological Q-waves have duration ≥0,03 sec and/or amplitude ≥25% of the R-wave amplitude. Pathological Q-waves must exist in at least two anatomically contiguous leads (i.e neighboring leads, such as aVF and III, or V4 and V5) in order to reflect an actual morphological abnormality. The existence of pathological Q-waves in two contiguous leads is sufficient for a diagnosis of Q-wave infarction. This is illustrated in **Figure 11**.

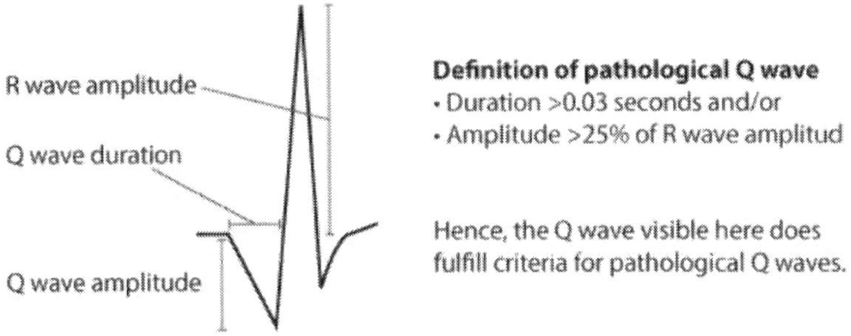

Figure 11. Criteria for pathological Q-waves.

Normal variants of Q-waves

Septal q-waves are small q-waves frequently seen in the lateral leads (V5, V6, aVL, I). They are due to the normal depolarization of the ventricular septum (see the previous discussion). Two small septal q-waves can actually be seen in V5–V6 in **Figure 10** (left-hand side).

An isolated and often large Q-wave is occasionally

seen in lead III. The amplitude of this Q-wave typically varies with ventilation and it is therefore referred to as a **respiratory Q-wave**. Note that the Q-wave must be isolated to lead III (i.e the neighboring lead, which is aVF, must not display a pathological Q-wave).

As noted above, the small r-wave in V1 is occasionally missing, which leaves a **QS-complex in V1** (a QRS complex consisting of only a Q-wave is referred to as a QS-complex). This is considered a normal finding provided that lead V2 shows an r-wave. If the R-wave is missing in lead V2 as well, then criteria for pathology is fulfilled (two QS-complexes).

Small Q-waves (which do not fulfill criteria for pathology) may be seen in all limb leads as well as V4–V6. If these Q-waves do not fulfill criteria for pathology, then they should be accepted. Leads V1–V3, on the other hand, should never display Q-waves (regardless of their size).

Abnormal (pathological) Q-waves

The most common cause of pathological Q-waves is myocardial infarction. If myocardial infarction leaves pathological Q-waves, it is referred to as Q-wave infarction. Criteria for such Q-waves are presented in Figure 11. Note that pathological Q-waves must exist in two anatomically contiguous leads.

Other causes of abnormal Q-waves are as follows:

- Left-sided pneumothorax
- Dextrocardia
- Perimyocarditis
- Cardiomyopathy
- Amyloidosis
- Bundle branch blocks, fascicular blocks
- Pre-excitation (WPW syndrome)
- Ventricular hypertrophy
- Acute corpulmonale

To differentiate these causes of abnormal Q-waves from Q-wave infarction, the following can be advised:

- If it is unlikely that the patient has coronary

heart disease, other causes are more likely. It should be noted, however, that up to 20% of Q-wave infarctions may develop without symptoms (The Framingham Heart Study).

- If coronary heart disease is likely, then infarction is the most probable cause of the Q-waves.
- The longer the Q-wave duration, the more likely that infarction is the cause of the Q-waves. Infarction Q-waves are typically >40 ms.

Examples of normal and pathological Q-waves (after acute myocardial infarction) are presented in Figure 12 below.

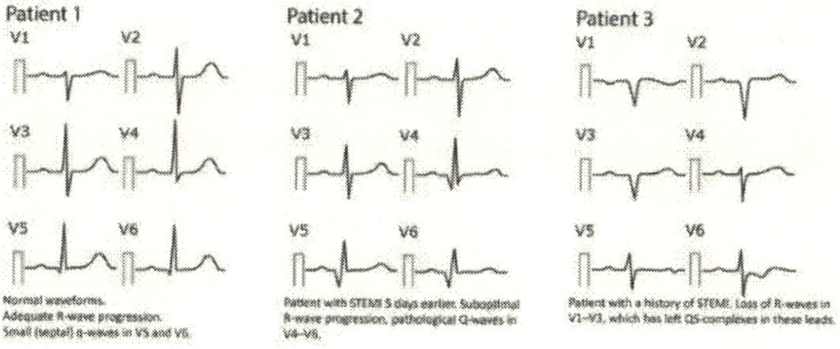

Figure 12. Normal and pathological Q-waves.

The ST segment: ST depression & ST elevation

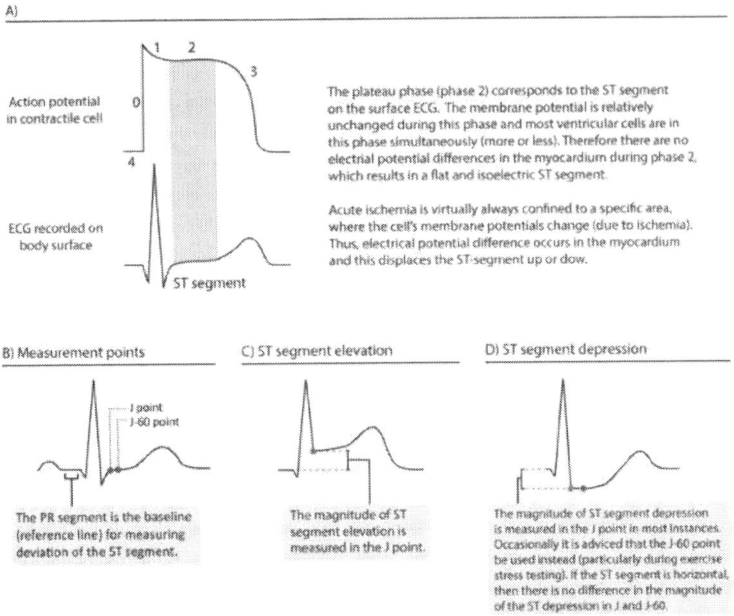

Figure 13. ST segment elevation and depression.

The ST segment corresponds to the plateau phase of the action potential (Figure 13). The ST segment extends from the J point to the onset of the T-wave. Because of the long duration of the plateau phase most contractile cells are in this phase at the same time (more or less). Moreover, the membrane potential is relatively unchanged during the plateau phase. These two factors are the reason why the ST segment is flat and isoelectric (i.e in level with the baseline).

Displacement of the ST segment is of fundamental importance, particularly in acute myocardial ischemia. Because myocardial ischemia affects a limited area and disturbs the cells' membrane potential (during phase 2), it engenders an electrical potential difference in the myocardium. The electrical potential difference exists between ischemic and normal myocardium and it results in displacement of the ST segment. The ST segment may be displaced upwards (ST segment elevation) or downwards (ST segment depression). The term ST segment deviation refers to elevation and depression of the ST segment. The magnitude of ST segment deviation is measured as the height difference (in millimeters) between the J point and the PR segment. Refer to **Figure 13** for examples.

Figure 14 below shows how to measure ST segment deviation.

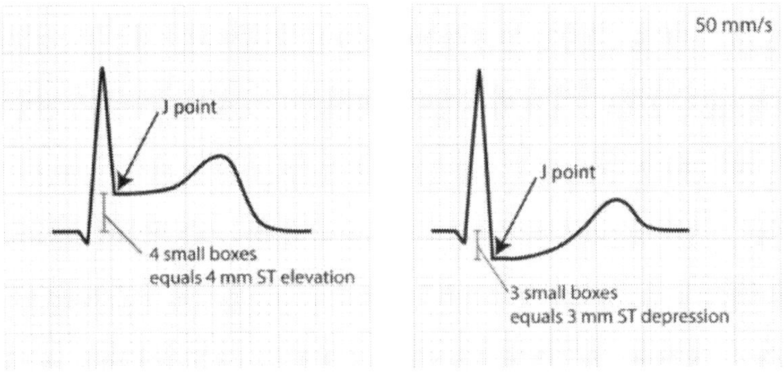

Figure 14. Example of measuring ST deviation (elevation and depression).

The following must be noted regarding the ST segment:

- The normal ST segment is flat and isoelectric. The transition from ST segment to T-wave is smooth, and not abrupt.
- ST segment deviation (elevation, depression) is measured as the height difference (in millimeters) between the J point and the baseline (the PR segment). ST segment deviation occurs in a wide range of conditions, particularly acute myocardial ischemia.
- Because the ST segment and the T-wave are electrophysiologically related, changes in the ST

segment are frequently accompanied by T-wave changes. The term ST-T segment changes (or simply ST-T changes) is used to refer to such ECG changes.

It must also be noted that the J point is occasionally suboptimal for measuring ST segment deviation. This is explained by the fact that the J point is not always isoelectric; this occurs if there are electrical potential differences in the myocardium by the end of the QRS complex (it typically causes J point depression). The reason for such electrical potential difference is that not all ventricular myocardial cells will finish their action potential simultaneously.

Myocardial cells which depolarized at the beginning of the QRS complex will not be in the exact same phase as cells which depolarized during the end of the QRS complex. Due to this, it is sometimes recommended that ST segment deviation be measured in the J-60 point, or J-80 point, which is located 60 and 80 milliseconds, respectively, after the J point (*Comprehensive Electrocardiology*, *MacFarlane et al*,

Springer, 2010; *Chou's Electrocardiologi*, *Surawicz*, *Elsevier 2010*).

At the time of J-60 and J-80, there is minimal chance that there are any electrical potential differences in the myocardium. Current guidelines, however, still recommend the use of the J point for assessing acute ischemia (Third Universal Definition of Myocardial Infarction, Thygesen et al, Circulation). A notable exception to this rule is the exercise stress test, in which the J-60 or J-80 is always used (because exercise frequently causes J point depression).

As mentioned above there are numerous other conditions that affect the ST-T segment and it is fundamental to be able to differentiate these. For this purpose, it is wise to subdivide ST-T changes into primary and secondary.

Primary and secondary ST-T changes

Primary ST-T changes are caused by **abnormal repolarization**. This is seen in ischemia, electrolyte disorders (calcium, potassium), tachycardia, increased sympathetic tone, drug side effects etc.

Secondary ST-T changes occur when **abnormal depolarization causes abnormal repolarization**. This is seen in bundle branch blocks (left and right bundle branch block), pre-excitation, ventricular hypertrophy, premature ventricular complexes, pacemaker stimulated beats etc. In each of these conditions, the depolarization is abnormal and this affects the repolarization so that it cannot be carried out normally.

The next discussion will be devoted to characterizing important and common ST-T changes.

ST segment depression

ST segment depression is measured in the J point. The reference point is, as usual, the PR segment. ST segment depression less than 0.5 mm is accepted in all leads. ST segment depression 0.5 mm or more is considered pathological. Some expert consensus documents also note that any ST segment depression in V2–V3 should be considered abnormal (because healthy individuals rarely display depressions in those leads). Please note that every cause of ST segment depression discussed below is illustrated in **Figure 15**. Study this figure carefully.

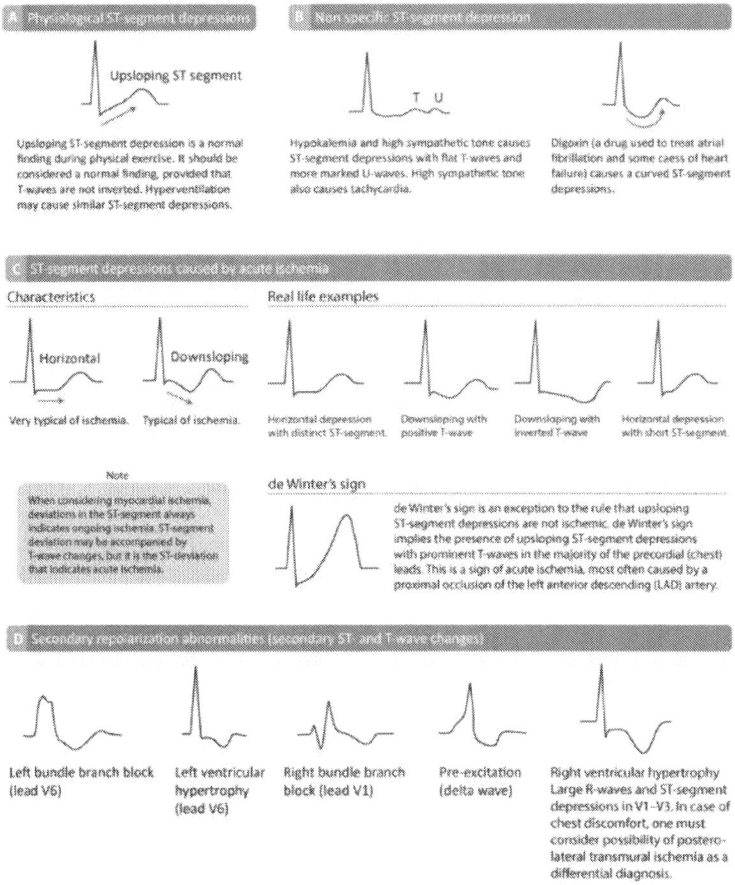

Figure 15. Various causes of ST segment depressions and their appearance.

Primary ST depressions

Physiological ST segment depressions occur during **physical exercise**. These ST segment depressions display an upsloping ST segment, typically depressed <1 mm in the J-60 point and the depressions are normalized rapidly after the exercise has ended. **Hyperventilation** brings about the same ST segment depressions as physical exercise. **Figure 15 A**.

Digoxin causes generalized ST segment depressions with a curved ST segment (generalized implies that the depression can be seen in most ECG leads). **Figure 15 B**.

Sympathetic tone and **hypokalemia** cause ST segment depressions (typically <0.5 mm).

Heart failure may cause ST segment depression in the left lateral leads (V5, V6, aVL and I) and these depressions are generally horizontal or downsloping.

Supraventricular tachycardias also cause ST segment depressions which typically occur in V4–V6 with a horizontal or slightly upsloping ST segment.

These ST segment depression should resolve within minutes after termination of the tachycardia.

Ischemic ST depressions display a horizontal or downsloping ST segment (this is a requirement according to North American and European guidelines). The horizontal ST segment depression is most typical of ischemia (Figure **15 C**). ST segment depressions with upsloping ST segments are rarely caused by myocardial ischemia. However, there is one notable exception, when an upsloping ST segment is actually caused by ischemia and the condition is actually alarming. Upsloping ST segment depressions which are accompanied by prominent T-waves in the majority of the precordial leads may be caused by acute occlusion of the left anterior descending coronary artery (LAD). This constellation – with upsloping ST depression and prominent T-waves in the precordial leads during chest discomfort – is referred to as **de Winters sign** (**Figure 15 C**).

Secondary ST depression

Secondary ST segment depressions occur in the

following conditions:

- Left ventricular hypertrophy
- Right ventricular hypertrophy
- Left bundle branch block
- Right bundle branch block
- Pre-excitation
- Pacemaker stimulation in the (right) ventricle

These are all common conditions in which an abnormal depolarization (altered QRS complex) causes abnormalities in the repolarization (altered ST-T segment). For example, a block in the left bundle branch means that the left ventricle will not be depolarized via the Purkinje network, but rather via the spread of the depolarization from the right ventricle. The abnormal ventricular depolarization will cause abnormal repolarization. these conditions are characterized by oppositely directed QRS- and ST-T-segments (recall that this is referred to as discordance). Hence, ECG leads with net positive QRS complexes will show ST segment depressions (as well as T-wave changes).

ECG changes in myocardial ischemia are discussed in section 3 (Acute & Chronic Myocardial Ischemia & Infarction) and a specific chapter discusses ST depression.

ST segment elevation

ST segment elevation is measured in the J-point. In the setting of chest discomfort (or other symptoms suggestive of myocardial ischemia) ST segment elevation is an alarming finding as it indicates that the ischemia is extensive and the risk of malignant arrhythmias is high. However, there are many other causes of ST segment elevations and for obvious reasons, one must be able to differentiate these. **Figure 16** displays characteristics of ischemic and non-ischemic ST segment elevations. This figure must also be studied in detail.

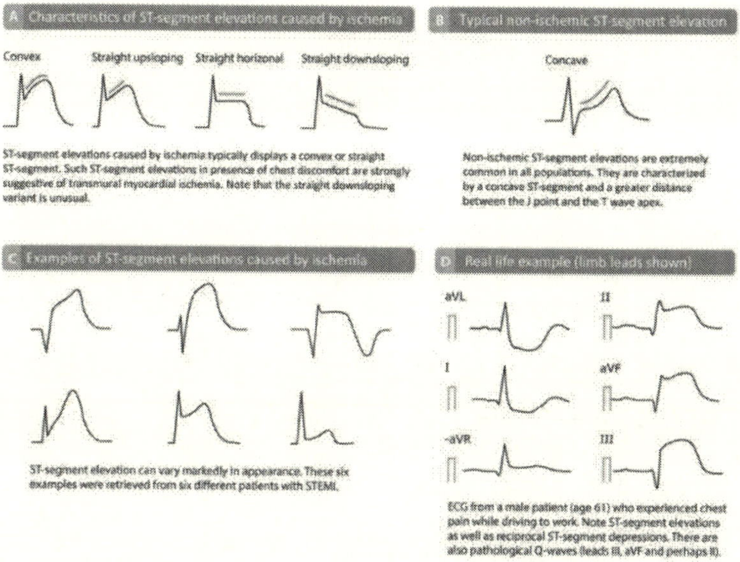

Figure 16. ST segment elevations.

Ischemia typically causes ST segment elevations with straight or convex ST segments (**Figure 16**, **panel A**). The straight ST segment can be either upsloping, horizontal or (rarely) downsloping. Non-ischemic ST segment elevations are typically concave (**Figure 16**, **panel B**). Concave ST segment elevations are extremely common in any population; e.g ST segment elevation in leads V2–V3 occur in 70% of all men under the age of 70.

There is no definite way to rule out myocardial

ischemia by judging the appearance of the ST segment, which is why North American and European guidelines assert that the appearance of the ST segment cannot be used to rule out ischemia.

The T-wave

Assessment of the T-wave represents a difficult but fundamental part of ECG interpretation. The normal T-wave in adults is positive in most precordial and limb leads. The T-wave amplitude is highest in V2–V3. The amplitude diminishes with increasing age. As noted above, the transition from the ST segment to the T-wave should be smooth. The T-wave is normally slightly asymmetric since its downslope (second half) is steeper than its upslope (first half). Women have a more symmetrical T-wave, a more distinct transition from ST segment to T-wave and lower T-wave amplitude.

The T-wave should be concordant with the QRS complex, meaning that a net positive QRS complex should be followed by a positive T-wave, and vice versa (**Figure 17**). Otherwise, there is discordance (opposite directions of QRS and T) which might be due to pathology. A negative T-wave is also called an inverted T-wave.

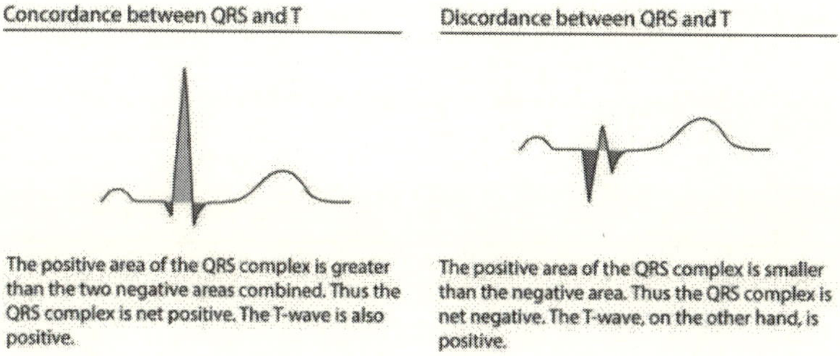

Figure 17. Discordance and concordance between QRS and ST-T.

T-wave changes are notoriously misinterpreted, particularly inverted T-waves. Below follows a discussion which aims to clarify some of the common misunderstandings. All T-waves are illustrated in **Figure 18**.

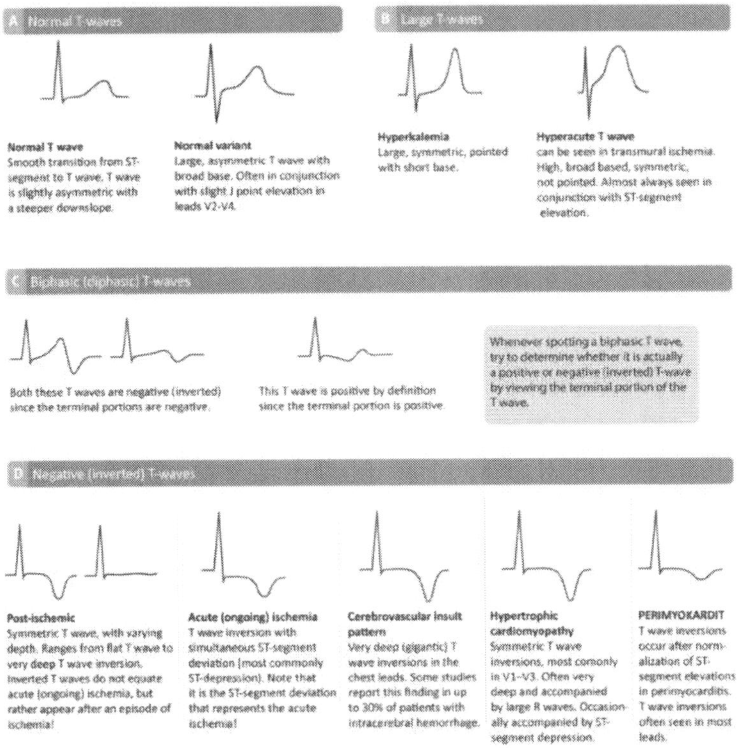

Figure 18. Normal and pathological T-waves.

Positive T-waves

Positive T-waves are rarely higher than 6 mm in the limb leads (typically highest in lead II). In the chest leads the amplitude is highest in V2–V3, where it may occasionally reach 10 mm in men and 8 mm in women. Usually, though, the amplitude in V2–V3 is around 6 mm and 3 mm in men and women, respectively. T-waves that are higher than 10 mm and

8 mm, in men and women, respectively, should be considered abnormal. A common cause of abnormally large T-waves is hyperkalemia, which results in high, pointed and asymmetric T-waves. These must be differentiated from hyperacute T-waves seen in the very early phase of myocardial ischemia. Hyperacute T-waves are broad-based, high and symmetric. Their duration is short; they typically disappear within minutes after a total occlusion in a coronary artery occurs (then of course, the ST segment will be elevated).

T-wave inversion (inverted / negative T-waves)

T-wave inversion means that the T-wave is negative. The T-wave is negative if its terminal portion is below the baseline, regardless of whether its other parts are above the baseline. T-wave inversions are frequently misunderstood, particularly in the setting of ischemia.

Normal T-wave inversion

An isolated (single) T-wave inversion in lead V1 is common and normal. It is generally concordant with the QRS complex (which is negative in lead V1). Isolated T-wave inversions also occur in leads V2, III or aVL. In any instance, one must verify whether the inversion is isolated, because if there is T-wave inversion in two anatomically contiguous leads, then it is pathological.

T-wave inversion in myocardial ischemia

Ischemia never causes isolated T-wave inversions. It is a general misunderstanding that T-wave inversions, without simultaneous ST-segment deviation, indicate acute (ongoing) myocardial ischemia. T-wave inversions without simultaneous ST-segment deviation are not ischemic! However, T-wave inversions that are accompanied by ST-segment deviation (either depression or elevation) is representative of ischemia (but in that scenario, it is actually the ST-segment deviation that signals that the ischemia is ongoing). Then one might wonder why T-wave inversions are included as criteria for myocardial infarction. This is explained by the fact that T-wave inversions do occur after an ischemic episode, and these T-wave inversions are referred to as *post-ischemic T-waves*. Such T-waves are seen after periods of ischemia, after infarction and after successful reperfusion (PCI).

Post-ischemic T-wave inversion is caused by abnormal repolarization. These T-wave inversions are symmetric with varying depth. They may be gigantic (10 mm or more) or less than 1 mm. Negative U-waves my occur when post-ischemic T-wave inversions are present. T-wave inversions may actually become chronic after myocardial infarction. Normalization of T-wave inversion after myocardial infarction is a good prognostic indicator. Please refer to Figure 37.

Secondary T-wave inversion

Secondary T-wave inversions – similar to secondary ST-segment depressions – are caused by bundle branch block, pre-excitation, hypertrophy, and ventricular pacemaker stimulation. T-wave inversions that are secondary to these conditions are typically symmetric and there is simultaneous ST-segment depression. Note that the T-wave inversion may actually persist for a period after normalization of the depolarization (if it occurs). This is referred to as T-wave memory or cardiac memory. Secondary T-wave inversions are illustrated in **Figure 19** (as well as **Figure 18 D**).

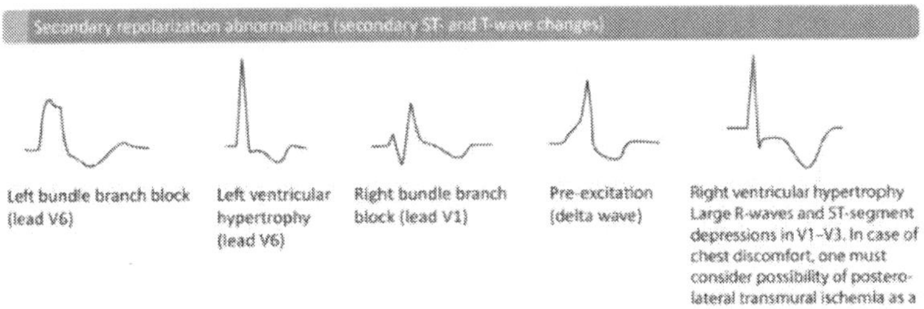

Figure 19. Secondary T-wave inversions.

Flat T-waves

T-waves with very low amplitude are common in the post-ischemic period. They are commonly seen in leads V1–V3 if the stenosis/occlusion is located in the left anterior descending artery. If the stenosis/occlusion is located in the left circumflex artery or right coronary artery, the flat T-waves are seen in leads II, aVF and III.

Biphasic (diphasic) T-waves

A biphasic T-wave has a positive and a negative deflection (Figure 37, panel C). It should be noted that the term "biphasic" is unfortunate because (1) biphasic T-waves carry no particular significance and (2) a T-wave is classified as positive or inverted based on its terminal portion; if the terminal portion is positive then the T-wave is positive and vice versa. Thus, a biphasic T-wave should be classified accordingly.

The T-waves in children and adolescents

The T-wave vector is directed to the left, downwards and to the back in children and adolescents. This explains why these individuals display T-wave inversions in the chest leads. T-wave inversions may be present in all chest leads. However, these inversions are normalized gradually during puberty. Some individuals may display persisting T-wave inversion in V1–V4, which is called *persisting juvenile T-wave pattern.* If all T-waves persist inverted into adulthood, the condition is referred to as *idiopathic global T-wave inversion.*

T-wave progression

T-wave progression follows the same rules as R-wave progression (see earlier discussion).

T-wave checklist

- I, II, -aVR, V5 and V6: should display positive T-waves in adults. aVR displays a negative T-wave.
- III and aVL: These leads occasionally display an isolated (single) T-wave inversion.
- aVF: positive T-wave, but occasionally flat.
- V1: Inverted or flat T-wave is rather common, particularly in women. The inversion is concordant with the QRS complex.
- V7–V9: should display a positive T-wave.

U-wave

A U-wave is occasionally seen after the T-wave. It is not known what engenders the U-wave. It is typically most prominent in leads V2–V3. young people, as well as athletes, have more prominent U-waves. Moreover, the U-wave is more prominent during slower heart rates. The height of the U-wave is typically one-third of the T-wave. Its first half is steeper than its second half.

U-wave inversion is rare but when seen, it is a strong indicator of pathology, particularly for ischemic heart disease and hypertension.

QT duration and corrected QT (QTc) duration

ECG interpretation always includes assessment of the QT (QTc) duration. The QT duration represents the total time for de- and repolarization. It is measured from the beginning of the QRS-complex to the end of the T-wave. Prolonged QT duration predisposes to life-threatening ventricular arrhythmias and therefore QT duration must always be assessed. Prolonged QT duration may either be congenital (genetic mutations, so-called long QT syndrome) or acquired (medications, electrolyte disorders). QT duration is inversely related to heart rate; QT duration increases at low heart rate and vice versa. Therefore one must adjust the QT duration for the heart rate, which yield corrected QT duration (Qtc). Bazett's formula has traditionally been used to calculate the corrected QT duration. The formula follows (all variables in seconds):

$$QTc = \frac{QT\ duration}{\sqrt{RR\ interval}}$$

Bazett's formula for calculating corrected QT duration (QTc).

Normal values for QTc interval

- Men: <0,450 seconds
- Women: <0,460 seconds

However, Bazett's formula is several decades old and has been questioned because it performs poorly at very low and very high heart rates. Newer formulas (which are incorporated in modern ECG machines) are to be preferred over Bazett's formula. QTc duration is calculated automatically in all modern ECG machines. The result is based on the lead with the longest QTc duration (typically leads V2–V3).

Causes of prolonged QTc duration:

antiarrhythmics (procainamide, disopyramide, amiodarone, sotalol), psychiatric medications (tricyclic antidepressants, SSRI, lithium etc); antibiotics (macrolides, kinolones, atovaquone, klorokine, amantadine, foscarnet, atazanavir); hypokalemia, hypocalcemia, hypomagnesemia; cerebrovascular insult (bleeding); myocardial ischemia; cardiomyopathy; bradycardia; hypothyroidism; hypothermia.

Short QTc syndrome (QTc <0,390 seconds) is uncommon and can be seen in hypocalcemia and during digoxin treatment. It is very rare but may cause malignant arrhythmias.

QT dispersion

The QT interval varies somewhat in the different leads. The difference between the shortest and the longest QT interval is the QT dispersion. Increased QT dispersion is associated with increased morbidity and mortality. This is presumably explained by a higher incidence of malignant ventricular arrhythmias. It has been suggested that the high risk of ventricular arrhythmias is due to vulnerability caused by marked local differences in the repolarization.

The electrical axis of the heart (heart axis)

Although often ignored, assessment of the electrical axis is an integral part of ECG interpretation. The electrical axis reflects the average direction of ventricular depolarization during ventricular contraction. The direction of the depolarization (and thus the electrical axis) is generally alongside the hearts longitudinal axis (to the left and downwards). Figure 20 shows the coordinate system where the green area displays the range of normal heart axis.

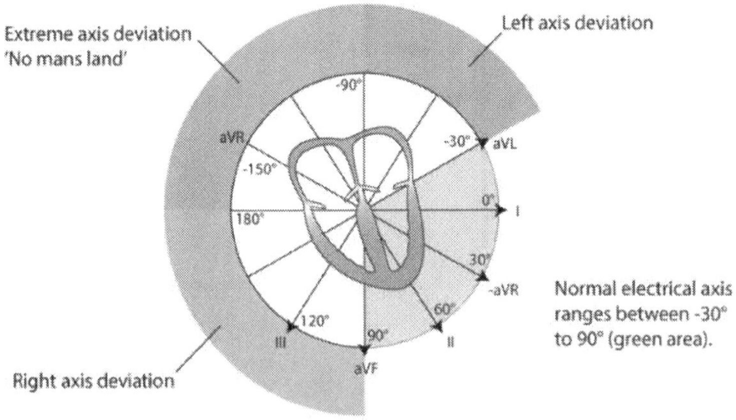

Figure 20. The electrical axis of the heart (heart axis).

As evident from the figure, the normal heart axis is between -30° and 90°. If the axis is more positive than 90° it is referred to as right axis deviation. If the axis is more negative than -30° it is referred to as left axis deviation. The axis is calculated (to the nearest degree) by the ECG machine. The axis can also be approximated manually by judging the net direction of the QRS complex in leads I and II. The following rules apply:

- Normal axis: Net positive QRS complex in leads I and II.
- Right axis deviation: Net negative QRS complex in lead I but positive in lead II.
- Left axis deviation: Net positive QRS complex in lead I but negative in lead II.
- Extreme axis deviation (-90°to 180°): Net negative QRS complex in leads I and II.

Axis deviation: right axis deviation (RAD) and left axis deviation (LAD)

Causes of right axis deviation

Normal in newborns. Right ventricular hypertrophy. Acute cor pulmonale (pulmonary embolism). Chronic cor pulmonale (COPD, pulmonary hypertension, pulmonary valve stenosis). Lateral ventricular infarction. Pre-excitation. Switched arm electrodes (negative P and QRS-T in lead I). Situs inversus. Left posterior fascicular block is diagnosed when the axis is between 90° and 180° with rS complex in I and aVL as well as qR complex in III and aVF (with QRS duration <0.12 seconds), provided that other causes of right axis deviation have been excluded.

Causes of left axis deviation

Left bundle branch block. Left ventricular hypertrophy. Inferior infarction. Pre-excitation. Left anterior fascicular block is diagnosed if the axis is between -45° and 90° with qR complex in aVL and QRS duration is 0,12 s, provided that other causes of left axis deviation have been excluded.

Causes of extreme axis deviation

Rare. Most likely due to misplaced limb electrodes. If

the rhythm is tachycardia with wide QRS complexes, then ventricular tachycardia is the most likely cause.

Chapter 6

Understanding The ECG Test

Once again let's define what an ECG/EKG is. An electrocardiogram (ECG) is a medical test that detects cardiac (heart) abnormalities by measuring the electrical activity generated by the heart as it contracts. The machine that records the patient's ECG is called an electrocardiograph.

The electrocardiograph records the electrical activity of the heart muscle and displays this data as a trace on a screen or on paper. This data is then interpreted by a medical practitioner.

ECGs from healthy hearts have a characteristic shape. Any irregularity in the heart rhythm or damage to the heart muscle can change the electrical activity of the heart so that the shape of the ECG is changed.

A doctor may recommend an ECG for people who may be at risk of heart disease because there is a family history of heart disease or because they smoke, are overweight, or have diabetes, high cholesterol or high blood pressure.

They may also recommend an ECG if a person is experiencing symptoms such as:

- chest pain
- shortness of breath
- dizziness
- fainting, or
- fast or irregular heartbeats (palpitations).

ECGs are often performed to monitor the health of people who have been diagnosed with heart problems, to help assess artificial cardiac pacemakers or to monitor the effects of certain medications on the heart.

The ECG procedure

There is no need to restrict food or drink before having an ECG test. Always let your doctor know what medications you are taking before you have an ECG, and if you have any allergies to adhesive tapes that may be used to attach electrodes.

When you go for an ECG test, you will need to

remove your upper clothing so that electrodes can be attached to your chest and limbs. (For women, wearing a separate top with trousers or a skirt can allow easy access to the chest.) The selected sites are shaved, if necessary.

Electrodes (sensors) are attached to the chest, arms and legs with suction cups or sticky gel. These electrodes detect the electrical currents generated by the heart – these are measured and recorded by the electrocardiograph.

The three major types of ECG are:

- **resting ECG** – you lie down for this type of ECG. No movement is allowed during the test, as electrical impulses generated by other muscles may interfere with those generated by your heart. This type of ECG usually takes 5 to 10 minutes
- **ambulatory ECG** – if you have an ambulatory or Holter ECG you wear a portable recording device for at least 24 hours. You are free to move around normally while the monitor is

attached. This type of ECG is used for people whose symptoms are intermittent (stop-start) and may not show up on a resting ECG, and for people recovering from heart attack to ensure that their heart is functioning properly. You record your symptoms in a diary, and note when they occur so that your own experience can be compared with the ECG

- **cardiac stress test** – this test is used to record your ECG while you ride on an exercise bike or walk on a treadmill. This type of ECG takes about 15 to 30 minutes to complete.

Immediately after an ECG procedure

When the procedure is completed, the electrodes are removed. An ECG is completely painless and non-invasive, as the skin is not penetrated. The doctor can interpret the results of your ECG straight away based on your medical history, symptoms and clinical examination.

Possible complications of an ECG

The ECG is a safe procedure with no known risks. It

does not send electric current to the body. Some people may be allergic or sensitive to the electrodes, which can cause local skin reddening.

Taking care of yourself at home after an ECG

After an ECG you can resume normal activities immediately. An ECG is non-invasive and doesn't involve medications (such as anaesthetics) or require recovery time.

Long-term outlook – heart problems diagnosed by ECG

The results of your ECG will determine what treatment you need, if any.

Some of the various heart problems that can be diagnosed by ECG include:

- enlargement of the heart
- congenital heart defects involving the conducting (electrical) system
- abnormal rhythm (arrhythmia) - rapid, slow or irregular heart beats
- damage to the heart such as when one of the heart's arteries is blocked (coronary occlusion)

- poor blood supply to the heart
- abnormal position of the heart
- heart inflammation - pericarditis or myocarditis
- cardiac arrest during emergency room or intensive care monitoring
- disturbances of the heart's conducting system
- imbalances in the blood chemicals (electrolytes) that control heart activity previous heart attacks.

A person with heart disease may have a normal ECG result if the condition does not cause a disturbance in the electrical activity of the heart. Other diagnostic methods may be recommended if heart disease is suspected.

Treatment for a heart condition depends on the diagnosed condition but may include:

- medication
- surgery
- dietary changes
- quitting smoking
- regular exercise.

For example, the following conditions diagnosed by ECG may require the treatment specified:

- disturbances in heart rhythm – medication or surgery (such as installing an artificial pacemaker)
- coronary artery disease or heart attack – medications, stenting, quitting cigarettes, dietary changes and coronary artery bypass surgery
- high blood pressure – dietary changes, regular exercise and medications.

Other tests for heart problems

Other tests that help diagnose heart problems include:

- physical examination
- chest x-rays
- echocardiogram (ultrasound of the heart)
- magnetic resonance imaging (MRI) or computerized tomography (CT) scans of the chest
- blood tests

- cardiac catheterization (insertion of a catheter through the blood vessels of the groin or wrist into the heart).

Chapter 7

NCLEX PRACTICE TEST QUESTIONS

1. A client has just undergone an electrocardiogram (ECG), the nurse notes that the QRS complex is measured to be 0.09 seconds. What is the first action the nurse should take?

Possible Answers:

A. Call the physician
B. Administer oxygen
C. Administer dopamine
D. Place on a cardiac monitor to check for arrhythmias

Correct answer: The nurse should document this finding

Explanation: This is a normal finding; the QRS should have duration between 0.6-0.12 seconds.

2. You are taking care of an elderly patient who is hospitalized for sudden onset of severe, diffuse abdominal pain out of proportion to the patient's abdominal physical exam that is also accompanied by rectal bleeding and palpitations. You obtain an ECG and notice a tachycardia, irregularly irregular rhythm without any distinct P waves. Which of the following is the most likely cardiac rhythm seen on this patient's ECG?

Possible Answers:

A. First-degree heart block
B. Sick sinus syndrome
C. Complete heart block
D. Atrial flutter
E. Atrial fibrillation (A-fib)

Correct answer: Atrial fibrillation (A-fib)

Explanation: The most likely cardiac rhythm on this patient's ECG is **atrial fibrillation**.

Atrial fibrillation is a tachyarrhythmia that is characterized on ECG by absence of distinct P waves, oscillating "f" waves that cause an irregular baseline rhythm, and abnormal, inconsistent R-R intervals that produce an **irregularly irregular rhythm**.

When a patient is in atrial fibrillation, the patient may be asymptomatic, but at other times, the patient may complain of a rapid heartbeat, or a feeling of uneasiness. The clues in this case that the patient is in atrial fibrillation are that the ECG shows the characteristic irregularly irregular rhythm, with an absence of any distinct P waves.

Clinically, the other clues are that the patient is complaining of palpitations while simultaneously experiencing sudden onset of severe, diffuse abdominal pain that is out of proportion to the abdominal physical exam, and is accompanied by rectal bleeding. This is very consistent with mesenteric ischemia (a condition in which a patient, **typically in atrial fibrillation**, projects a blood clot to one of the mesenteric vessels, causing ischemia to the bowel served by the affected vessel). While, this was not asked in the question explicitly, and the question could be answered without this knowledge, this helps confirm the diagnosis if you are aware of it.

The other answers are incorrect for the following

reasons:

A. Atrial flutter typically presents with a "sawtooth" waveform and has more regularity in wavelength.

B. Sick sinus syndrome is also known as tachy-brady syndrome, indicating that the patient has frequent fluctuations between tachycardia and bradycardia. In this instance, we have ECG findings that are very consistent with atrial fibrillation and show no evidence of bradycardia.

C. First-degree heart block and complete heart block are each typically characterized by bradycardia rather than tachycardia, and do not appear like atrial fibrillation on ECG.

3. A patient presents with thirty minute history of substernal chest pain that radiates to his left jaw. Which of the following EKG changes would you expect in this patient if his troponin level came back positive at 0.89$\frac{ng}{mL}$?

Possible Answers:

A. ST elevation

B. PR widening

C. PR shortening

D. QT prolongation

E. ST depression

Correct answer: ST elevation

Explanation: Substernal chest pain that radiates to the jaw is classic of myocardial infarction. Elevated troponin and EKG changes help confirm the diagnosis (reference levels are about 0.01ngmL. ST segment elevation is classically seen in myocardial infarctions that result in positive troponin.

4. You are a nurse taking care of a patient in the emergency room. Among other acute labwork and imaging, you obtain an electrocardiogram (ECG) of the patient. The ECG shows Osborn waves. Which of the following is the most common cause of Osborn waves on ECG?

Possible Answers:

A. Ethanol toxicity

B. Hypothermia

C. Carbon monoxide poisoning

D. Lead poisoning

E. Hyperthermia

Correct answer: Hypothermia

Explanation: The correct answer is "hypothermia." Osborn waves on electrocardiogram are the pathognomonic finding associated with hypothermia (to a core body temperature of lower than 32 C). Osborn waves are observed as upward deflections in the ECG reading between the QRS and ST intervals with an elevation at the S point (which is sometimes also referred to as the J point). While hypothermia is the most common cause of Osborn waves, they may also be observed in patients with coronary vasospasm, hypercalcemia, ventricular fibrillation, or brain trauma.

Neither hyperthermia, ethanol toxicity, carbon monoxide poisoning, nor lead poisoning are associated with Osborn waves on ECG.

5. An EKG of your patient shows peaked T-waves. This finding correlates to which electrolyte abnormality?

Possible Answers:

A. High calcium
B. High sodium
C. High potassium
D. Low potassium
E. Low sodium

Correct answer: High potassium

Explanation: Peaked T-waves are a warning sign for elevated levels of potassium in the body. On the other hand, flattened T-waves are potentially indicative of low levels of potassium. Hyperkalemia (high potassium) is a potentially dangerous condition that can lead to cardiac abnormalities and potentially death.

6. What is the most common EKG finding in a patient with a pulmonary embolism?

Possible Answers:

A. Sinus bradycardia

B. ST elevation

C. ST depression

D. Sinus tachycardia

Correct answer: Sinus tachycardia

Explanation: Sinus tachycardia is the most common EKG finding in a pulmonary embolism. This represents the heart beating faster as an infarction occurs within the lung tissue. Peaked T waves are seen in hyperkalemia. ST elevation is seen in myocardial infarction, and ST depression is seen in myocardial ischemia. Sinus bradycardia would not be the expected finding in a PE.

7. A 38-year-old female is brought to the Emergency Department with complaints of her "heart beating out of her chest". She is diaphoretic, tachypneic and her BP is 70/40. The cardiac monitor shows supraventricular tachycardia. Valsalva maneuvers and three doses of Adenosine have not been successful.

The nurse should immediately:

A. Prepare the patient for synchronized cardioversion.
B. Give Epinephrine 1 mg IV and repeat in 3 minutes.
C. Give Adenosine 6 mg IV per protocol.
D. Perform unilateral carotid massage.

Correct answer: Prepare the patient for synchronized cardioversion.

8. Prior to discharge from the Emergency Department, the nurse prints a rhythm strip on a patient and notices that the P wave cannot be detected and the QRS complex is 0.24 seconds. This is a change in the patient's condition. What is the best action for the nurse to take?

A. Measure the PR interval.
B. Prepare the patient for discharge.
C. Notify the physician of this abnormal strip.
D. Continue to monitor for abnormalities.

Correct answer: Notify the physician of this

abnormal strip.

Rationale:

c.) is correct because notifying the physician of the abnormal rhythm would be the most appropriate response. The patient has experienced a rhythm change and requires further treatment. a.) is not correct for measuring the PR would not be possible as there is no P wave present. Since the QRS interval and other parameters given are abnormal, discharging the patient would not be appropriate at this point.

b.) is not correct as discharging the patient is not appropriate or safe practice.

d.) is not correct because continuing to monitor the patient without any other actions would be inappropriate as the patient has experienced a change in condition.

9. A patient is to have synchronized cardioversion for treatment of atrial flutter. He has received Heparin 500 units subcutaneously. Which of the following interventions should now be performed?

A. Assist the MD in intubating the patient to stabilize airway.
B. Sedate the patient with Versed 2 mg IV push per protocol.
C. Set the defibrillator in asynchronous mode and charge to 300 joules.
D. Steadily increase the voltage until the beats are captured.

Correct answer: Sedate the patient with Versed 2 mg IV push per protocol.

Rationale:

b.) is correct since cardioversion is very painful, the patient should be sedated prior to the procedure.

a.) is not correct as intubation is usually not indicated prior to cardioversion.

c.) is not correct as synchronized cardioversion is performed at less voltage than defibrillation (360 joules). The defibrillator should be set in synchronous mode so the shock will be delivered on the R wave.

d.) is not correct because steadily increasing the voltage until the beats are captured is indicative of pacemaker therapy and not synchronized cardioversion.

10. When a patient has long-term atrial fibrillation, the nurse would expect to include which drug in the plan of care to minimize the greatest risk that is commonly associated with atrial fibrillation?

A. Beta blockers

B. Digitalis

C. Anticoagulants

D. Antiarrhythmics

Correct answer: Anticoagulants

Rationale:

c.) is correct because it reflects the greatest risk or complication of thrombi or emboli that occurs with long-term atrial fibrillation. Coumadin is often given prophylactically to prevent stroke, clots, or emboli from developing when hospitalizing a patient with long-term atrial fibrillation.

11. The nurse should understand that which of the following treatments for Second Degree Type II AV Block would be appropriate?

(Select all that apply)

A. Temporary pacemaker insertion
B. Close monitoring without intervention
C. Atropine to increase heart rate if symptomatic
D. Coronary stent placement to improve blood flow to myocardium
E. An implantable defibrillator surgically implanted

Correct answer:

a.) Temporary pacemaker insertion

c.) Atropine to increase heart rate if symptomatic

d.) Coronary stent placement to improve blood flow to myocardium

Rationale: a, c, and d are correct. Temporary

pacing may be needed and atropine will temporarily improve heart rate cardiac output until the pacemaker can be inserted.

b.) is incorrect because Type II has a tendency to develop complete heart block where adequate cardiac output is not maintained and arrest is likely. Type I can be monitored and minimal treatment is needed unless unstable hemodynamics are present.

e.) is incorrect because a defibrillator is not called for since it is the ventricle that is trying to maintain the cardiac output from the decreased conduction between the atria and the ventricles. An implanted pacemaker may be needed permanently.

12. The nurse would expect which of the following to be the first choice to treat a stable patient with ventricular tachycardia?

A. Amiodarone

B. Procainamide

C. Synchronized cardioversion

D. Atropine

Correct answer: Amiodarone

13. A 21-year-old female is seen in the Emergency Department for vomiting and diarrhea for 3 days. Her BP is 94/64 and her EKG rhythm shows that she is sinus tachycardia. The best action for the nurse to take initially is to:

A. Request pain medication for the patient.
B. Cardiovert the patient immediately.
C. Give Adenosine 6 mg IV push.
D. Start IV and bolus normal saline per protocol.

Correct answer: Start IV and bolus normal saline per protocol

Rationale:

d.) is correct because the patient is dehydrated due to vomiting and diarrhea and needs IV fluids. The rhythm strip is sinus tachycardia and the cause is treated.

a.) is not correct because no information is given regarding the presence of pain.
b.) is not correct because Cardioversion is not an

appropriate action for sinus tachycardia.

c.) is not correct because Adenosine is only given for SVT.

About the Author

Amanda Caldwell is a registered Nurse working in oncology. She attended Gordon State College where she got a Bachelor's degree 2014 and a Master's degree at Georgia College & State University in 2019.

She has a passion for teaching and nursing and her goal is to create a generation of highly skilled and educated nurses. She so much loves explaining complicated things in simple ways, and her writing is a true reflection of what she loves.

Made in the USA
Middletown, DE
26 September 2020

20631755R00104